Workbook

American Red Cross: Adult CPR

ISBN: 0-86536-075-8

Acknowledgments

This course is based on the standards and guidelines published by the 1985 National Conference on Cardiopulmonary Resuscitation (CPR) and Emergency Cardiac Care (ECC). Recommendations of the National Academy of Sciences-National Research Council Committee to Advise the American National Red Cross were also used in the development of this course. The NAS-NRC committee, under the chairmanship of George T. Anast, M.D., has continued to advise the American Red Cross, providing a channel for extending the first aid and emergency response recommendations of the medical profession to the American public.

The course and this book were designed and written by Allan Braslow, Ph.D., with technical and instructional design assistance from David J. Lindstrom and William J. Schneiderman. Dr. Braslow served as faculty at the 1985 National Conference on CPR and Emergency Cardiac Care, and has served as University Advisor on Emergency Medical Services for the University of Illinois.

Technical advice and review were provided by Michael L. Angell, Greater Rhode Island Chapter; Glenn R. Blafield, Greater Carolinas Chapter; Donald R. Workman, Central Florida Chapter; Nancy S. Ludlow, Western Operations Headquarters; and C.P. Dail and John M. Malatak, national headquarters. Thanks are also extended to the following Red Cross chapters that assisted in testing this course: Greater Carolinas Chapter, Charlotte, N.C.; Greater Hartford Chapter, Farmington, Conn.; Palo Alto Chapter, Palo Alto, Calif.; Greater Rhode Island Chapter, Providence, R.I.; Sacramento Area Chapter, Sacramento, Calif.; and the District of Columbia Chapter, Washington, D.C.

Field representatives providing advice and guidance were:

Norman G. Bottenberg, Seattle-King County Chapter, Seattle, Wash.

Frank Carroll, District of Columbia Chapter, Washington, D.C.

Raymond A. Cranston, Farmington Hills, Mich.

Gerald M. Dworkin, Springfield, Va.

Diana M. Meyer, Greater Hartford Chapter, Farmington, Conn.

William R. Murphy, Jr., Indianapolis, Ind.

Margaret E. Neill, Portland, Oreg.

Gary D. Sullivan, Mile High Chapter, Denver, Colo.

Acknowledgments

Technical review of this manuscript was provided by the following experts in emergency medical services and emergency cardiac care:

George T. Anast, M.D., Chairman, NAS-NRC Committee to Advise the American National Red Cross; Northern Wisconsin Orthopedic Center, Woodruff, Wis.

Leon Chameides, M.D., Director of Pediatric Cardiology, Clinical Professor of Pediatrics, University of Connecticut Health Center, Hartford Hospital, Hartford, Conn.

Gail Cooper, Chief, Emergency Medical Services, County of San Diego, Calif.

Judith Donegan, M.D., Ph.D., Chairperson of the AHA Subcommittee on Emergency Cardiac Care; Professor of Anesthesia, University of California, San Francisco, Calif.

John Field, M.D., Chief, Division of Emergency Medicine; Director, Emergency Medical Services, Milton S. Hershey Medical Center, Pennsylvania State University, Hershey, Pa.

Benjamin Honigman, M.D., Director, Emergency Department, University of Colorado Health Sciences Center, Denver, Colo.

David J. Lindstrom, M.A., Director, Office of Emergency Medical Services, Pennsylvania State University, University Park, Pa.

George E. Membrino, Ph.D., Associate Dean for Continuing Education, and Associate Professor, Department of Family and Community Medicine, University of Massachusetts Medical Center, Worcester, Mass.

William J. Schneiderman, Adjunct Clinical Instructor, NYU/Bellevue Hospital Center, Emergency Care Institute, and former Education Coordinator, Department of Emergency Medical Services, New York Infirmary-Beekman Downtown Hospital, New York, N.Y.

This book is dedicated to the thousands of volunteers who contribute their time and talents to teach lifesaving skills to the American public, and to the memory of Donald A. Sleeper, former assistant national director of first aid for the American Red Cross.

Contents

Contents

About This Course

Why the American Red Cross Teaches This Course

This year about a million and a half people in the United States will have heart attacks. One third of these people will die. **This means that about 1,500 people die every day from heart attacks.**

Most victims who die from a heart attack die before ever reaching a hospital. But some survive because a bystander trained in the skills taught in this course knew what to do and because his or her community had an emergency medical services (EMS) system to provide advanced care at the scene of the emergency.

One out of every two people in the United States can expect to die from a heart attack or a related disease of the blood vessels. This is an important national problem. In an effort to reduce this death toll, the American Red Cross has developed this **Adult CPR** course. This course will teach you:

1. How to reduce your risk of dying from a heart attack.
2. How to recognize the signals of a heart attack and give first aid in order to reduce the chances that a person's heart will stop.
3. How to provide CPR (cardiopulmonary resuscitation) to keep the brain and heart of a cardiac arrest victim supplied with oxygen until advanced medical help arrives.
4. How to give first aid for choking and other breathing emergencies that could lead to cardiac arrest.
5. How to use your community's emergency medical services (EMS) system effectively.

This course has been designed to teach you lifesaving skills. We want you to learn as much as you can about heart attacks, CPR, and respiratory emergencies. Your desire to learn the material is the key to success.

About This Course

Workbook

This book includes several things to help you get the most out of this course.

Objectives

Each chapter in this book begins with a list of objectives. The objectives tell you what you will learn in that chapter.

Review Questions

Throughout each chapter you will find review questions. Answering these questions will help you check how well you are learning and will prepare you for the final test. Write your answers in the book. The correct answers follow each group of review questions, so be sure to go back and correct your answers. Change any wrong answers.

Skill Sheets

Some chapters include skill sheets with checklists that describe how to perform certain first aid skills. You will use these when you practice the skills you will be learning in the course. You will be practicing on a partner and on a manikin.

Glossary

A glossary has been included at the end of this book to explain words that you may not know.

Films

In some versions of this course, you will also see some short films. These show real-life situations in which you would use the skills learned in this course. These films contain demonstrations of the skills you will be practicing. Watching the demonstrations closely will help you do well in the practice sessions.

Tests

There are two types of tests in this course: **skill tests** and a **written test.** Skill tests are given after you have practiced a skill and are ready to be tested.

A 25-question written test will be given at the end of the course. This is a multiple-choice test about the things you have learned in this course.

How Much Do You Know About Heart Attacks and CPR?

Here are some questions about CPR, heart attacks, and breathing emergencies. These questions should help you think about your role in dealing with and preventing the types of emergencies covered in this class. **Check the best answer.** Don't expect to be able to answer every question.

1. When someone has a heart attack, people often think of the attack as a sudden event. Later in this course you will learn that most heart attacks are caused by a disease. At what age do you think the **disease** that causes heart attacks begins?
   - ☐ Heart disease begins around the age of 30.
   - ☐ Heart disease can begin in early childhood.

2. If you want to reduce your risk of having a heart attack, how can you do it?
   - ☐ You can reduce your risk of having a heart attack by having your blood pressure checked regularly, giving up smoking, and watching what you eat.
   - ☐ There is no way to reduce your risk of a heart attack.

3. Which of the following is a common signal of a heart attack?
   - ☐ A person having a heart attack may have pain or pressure in the chest.
   - ☐ A person having a heart attack may complain of pain in the legs.

4. What does CPR do?
   - ☐ It restarts the heart of a heart attack victim.
   - ☐ It supplies oxygen to the body's cells when a person's heart has stopped beating.

5. You arrive for work in the morning and find one of your friends lying on the floor. He is motionless and lying on his back. You kneel down, tap him on the shoulder, and ask him if he's OK. He doesn't answer you. You shout for help. What do you think a trained person would do next?

☐ Check to see if the person is breathing and has a pulse.

☐ Check for a medical ID bracelet that would tell what might be wrong.

6. What should you do for someone who is coughing hard and seems to have something caught in the throat?

☐ Stay with the person, but do not interfere with the person's attempts to cough up the object.

☐ Offer a glass of water and instruct the person to drink it slowly.

Answers

1. **Heart disease can begin in early childhood.**
   Scientists think that cardiovascular disease, the disease that causes heart attacks, begins early in life, perhaps in early childhood. Studies have shown that some 19-year-olds already have partially clogged arteries that could cause heart attacks later in life.

2. **You can reduce your risk of a heart attack by having your blood pressure checked regularly, giving up smoking, and watching what you eat.**
   These are three good ways of lowering your risk of having a heart attack, but there are more. In this course you will learn what causes heart attacks and what can be done to reduce the risk of dying from a heart attack.

3. **A person having a heart attack may have pain or pressure in the chest.**
   The most significant signal of a heart attack is pain and/or pressure in the chest. Other signals of a heart attack include sweating, nausea, and shortness of breath. Heart attack victims often try to deny the fact that they are having a heart attack. For this reason, being able to recognize that a person is having a heart attack is one very important skill that you will learn in this course. If you recognize a heart attack early, the victim's chances of surviving can be greatly improved.

4. **CPR supplies oxygen to the body's cells when a person's heart has stopped beating.**
   CPR is a way of supplying oxygen to the body's cells when a person's heart has stopped (cardiac arrest). It works because you can breathe air into the victim's lungs to get oxygen into the blood. Then, when you press on the chest, you move oxygen-carrying blood through the body. While many people think that CPR alone can save a victim of cardiac arrest by restarting the heart, it is really more complicated than that. It takes immediate CPR combined with the delivery of advanced medical care within a short time, generally eight to ten minutes, to give the victim the best chance of survival. When CPR is combined with quick delivery of the right medical care, it has been

shown that about 40 percent of victims of cardiac arrest can be saved. CPR is used to keep the cells of the victim's body from dying until more advanced medical help arrives.

5. **Check to see if the person is breathing and has a pulse.**

   You must check the victim for the most serious problems first, and deal with these problems immediately to increase the victim's chances of survival. The emergency action principles that you will learn in this course will give you the steps that you should follow for dealing with emergency situations.

6. **Stay with the person, but do not interfere with the person's attempts to cough up the object.**

   If the person is coughing hard, he or she is also breathing. In that case, you should let the person try to cough up the object. In this course you will learn how to tell if a person who is choking needs your help, and what to do to clear the airway.

1 What This Course Will Teach You

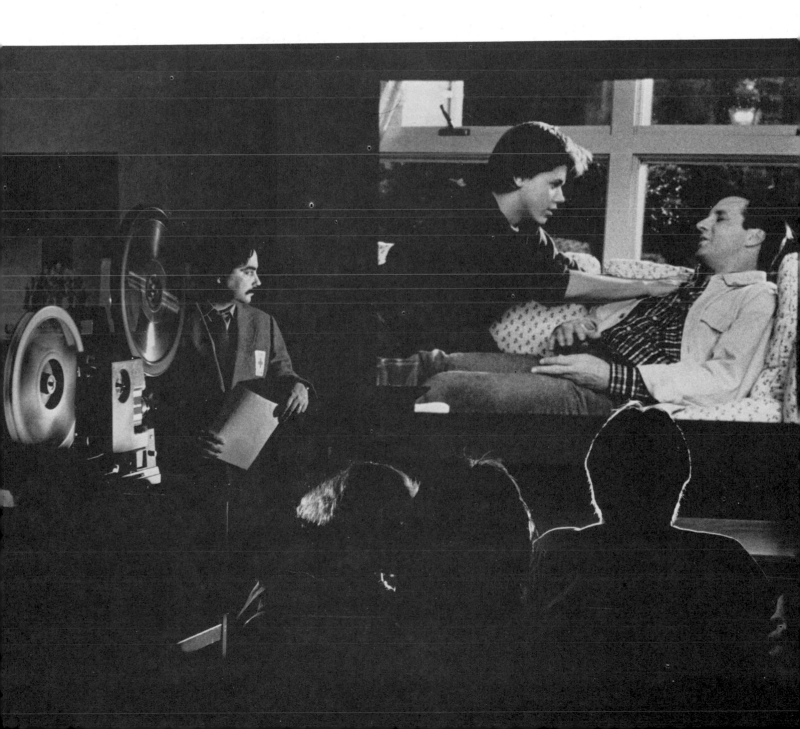

You are visiting your cousin, David, and his wife, Ann. The three of you have just finished eating and are sitting in the backyard. After a few minutes, David stops talking.

"Are you feeling all right?" Ann asks.

"Sure, I'm OK," David says.

"Well, you don't look very OK to me," Ann replies.

"I had a little indigestion just before we ate and I took something for it," he explains, "but it doesn't seem to be doing much good."

David is having a heart attack. His heart muscle is dying, making it difficult and painful for his heart to pump blood.

A moment later, David collapses. He is not breathing and his heart has stopped beating — he is in **cardiac arrest.** Someone must help David immediately.

Two things must happen if David is to be given the best chance to live. CPR must be started right away, and advanced emergency medical care must get to David within eight to ten minutes.

David may be lucky if there is a CPR-trained bystander and his community has ambulances staffed with personnel trained to give advanced care. If David does not get prompt CPR and advanced care, it is unlikely that he will survive.

Would YOU Know What To Do?

In this course you will learn what to do for heart attacks and what you can do to prevent heart attacks from happening. You will also learn how to begin care for a cardiac arrest victim by performing CPR and how to give first aid for choking and other breathing emergencies that could lead to cardiac arrest.

Objectives

By the time you finish reading this chapter, you should be able to do the following:

1. Name the three leading causes of death in the United States.
2. Explain how to reduce the chance of death from heart attack.
3. Explain the purpose of CPR.
4. Describe what is needed to save the life of a victim of cardiac arrest.
5. Describe the citizen's role as part of the emergency medical services (EMS) system.

Heart Disease Is the Number One Killer

Cardiovascular disease, disease of the heart and blood vessels, is the leading cause of death in the United States. Cancer is the second leading cause of death. The third leading cause is injury, of which automobile-related injuries are the most common *(Fig. 1)*.

Overall, one in every five Americans has some form of cardiovascular disease. Or, put another way, one out of every five participants in this class is likely to have cardiovascular disease.

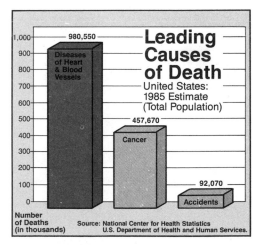

Figure 1
Leading Causes of Death

Reducing Deaths From Heart Attacks

Most people who die of a heart attack die before they ever reach a hospital. The best way to reduce deaths from heart attacks and cardiovascular disease is not simply to equip every hospital with the latest equipment and trained specialists, but to try to prevent the disease that causes heart attacks.

Many people believe that a heart attack occurs suddenly and by chance. This is rarely true. The disease that most often causes heart attacks (cardiovascular disease) is believed to begin in early childhood. The disease gets worse as we get older. As it gets worse, the chance of having a heart attack increases.

Preventing cardiovascular disease involves knowing what things increase your chances of having a heart attack, and knowing what you can do to control these things.

Preventing death when a heart attack does occur involves recognizing the signals of a heart attack and knowing what to do. These topics will be discussed in more detail later in this course.

Most people who die of a heart attack die within two hours of the time when the heart attack signals start. Some victims die before anyone recognizes the need for emergency medical care. In order to save the lives of heart attack victims, emergency care must be immediately available in the community when the heart attack happens. This emergency care depends on citizens' being able to recognize the signals of a heart attack, provide first aid, and call for emergency medical services. Your being able to recognize the signals of a heart attack, and acting quickly before the heart stops, can mean the difference between life and death for many victims.

But if a person's heart has stopped (cardiac arrest), CPR is needed to keep oxygen-carrying blood flowing from the lungs to the brain and heart until more advanced emergency medical care arrives. The bystander who is able to give that lifesaving care could be you. Some experts estimate that if all victims of cardiac arrest received prompt CPR, followed by advanced medical care within 8 to 10 minutes, many victims could be saved *(Fig. 2)*.

There are other situations, in addition to heart attack, that can lead to cardiac arrest and the need for CPR. For example, victims of drowning, electrocution, drug overdose, and

• Victim's Heart Stops

ZERO MINUTES

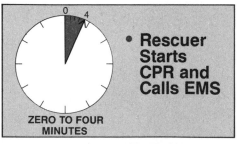

• Rescuer Starts CPR and Calls EMS

ZERO TO FOUR MINUTES

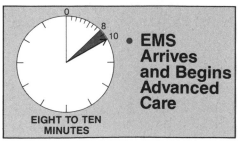

• EMS Arrives and Begins Advanced Care

EIGHT TO TEN MINUTES

Figure 2
Critical Times for Saving a Life

poisoning may go into cardiac arrest. If a person's heart stops for any reason, CPR must be started immediately and advanced medical help must arrive within 8 to 10 minutes. You should also know that sometimes the heart just stops without warning.

Your Role

Rescuers—citizens like you—play a vital role both in preventing heart attacks from happening and in acting to give first aid when they do happen. When a heart attack or other cardiac emergency occurs, it is up to you to recognize that emergency medical help is needed, to begin first aid, and to alert your community's emergency medical services (EMS) system. In some situations, this can be done before a heart attack turns into a cardiac arrest. Should cardiac arrest occur, you can use CPR to keep the brain and body cells supplied with oxygen during the critical minutes that it takes for advanced medical help to reach the victim.

Review Questions

Check the best answer and fill in the blanks with the right word(s).

1. List the three leading causes of death in the United States.

    1) _____

    2) _____

    3) _____

2. When does the disease that causes heart attack begin?
    ☐ a. Cardiovascular disease usually begins around the age of 50.
    ☐ b. Cardiovascular disease begins around the age of 30.
    ☐ c. Cardiovascular disease can begin in early childhood.

3. Assuming that CPR is started immediately after a cardiac arrest, how soon must a victim receive advanced medical care to have the best chance of survival?
    ☐ a. Within 8 to 10 minutes.
    ☐ b. Within 30 minutes.
    ☐ c. Within an hour.

Answers

1. The three leading causes of death are:

   1) **Cardiovascular disease**
   2) **Cancer**
   3) **Injuries**

2. c. **Cardiovascular disease can begin in early childhood.**

3. a. A victim of cardiac arrest must receive advanced medical care **within 8 to 10 minutes** to have the best chance of survival.

Now let's return for a moment to the example given at the beginning of this chapter. If you had been trained in first aid, what could you have done to save David's life?

After David collapsed, you could have checked for breathing and pulse. You could have started CPR while telling someone to phone for emergency medical help. You could have then continued to give CPR until advanced medical care arrived.

But there is something even more effective that you, as a trained rescuer, might have done. By recognizing the signals of a heart attack, you might have realized during dinner that something was seriously wrong with David. You then could have started first aid and called your community's emergency medical services system for help. Advanced medical care might have reached David before his heart stopped beating.

2

How to Deal With an Emergency (Emergency Action Principles)

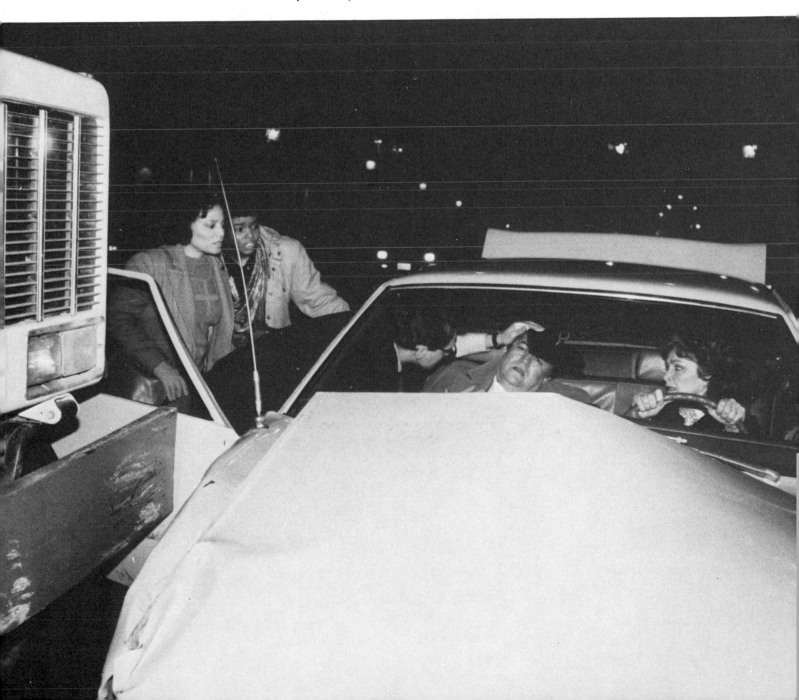

The next few chapters will tell you what to do for respiratory emergencies, choking, heart attacks, and cardiac arrest. You will also learn about how these emergencies can be prevented. But before you learn about first aid for these emergencies, you should know about certain actions that should be taken in **every** emergency situation. These are called **emergency action principles.**

Objectives

By the time you finish reading this chapter, you should be able to do the following:

1. List the four steps of the emergency action principles (the four actions that should be taken in every emergency).
2. Describe why it is important to follow the same basic steps in **every** emergency situation.
3. Describe why it is important to identify yourself to the victim and bystanders.
4. Describe the chief purpose of the **primary survey.**
5. Describe the steps of the primary survey.
6. Explain why you should complete the primary survey before phoning the emergency medical services system (EMS) for help.
7. List at least four pieces of information you should give an EMS dispatcher when phoning for help.
8. Describe the chief purpose of the **secondary survey.**
9. Describe the steps of the secondary survey.
10. Describe why it is important to ask for permission from a conscious person before beginning first aid.

Emergency Action Principles

This chapter will give you a four-step plan of action for emergency situations. You should follow these steps so that you don't forget anything that might affect personal safety (yours and the victim's) and the victim's survival. To see why emergency action principles are needed, think about the following situation:

You are sitting at home watching television when you hear a cry for help from outside. You run out of the house and see a man lying face down on the side of the road. What do you do?

Most people would run straight to the man. But think for a moment. Is there anything wrong with doing that? Is there something you might miss if you ran straight to the victim?

Could there be another victim, one who is more seriously injured? Could a quick look around give you an idea of what happened and what injuries the person might have? Could the situation be dangerous to you and others nearby?

How to Deal With an Emergency (Emergency Action Principles)

If you run straight to the victim and begin to deal with the first problem you see, many things could go wrong. You could become injured too. Also, other victims could be overlooked. Minor injuries might be taken care of before major ones. People at the scene might assume that someone else had called the emergency medical services (EMS) system for help. A trained rescuer should have a plan of action to handle emergency situations. Here are the four steps of the emergency action principles. They should always be performed in this order. They are explained in the rest of this chapter.

1. Survey the scene.
2. Do a primary survey of the victim.
3. Phone the emergency medical services (EMS) system for help.
4. Do a secondary survey of the victim.

Review Questions

Fill in the blanks with the right word(s) or number.

1. It is important to follow the same basic steps in every emergency situation so that you don't forget anything that might affect _____ _____ (yours and the victim's) and the victim's _____.

2. Put the following four steps of the emergency action principles in the right order.

   Order

   _____ Phone the EMS system for help.

   _____ Survey the scene.

   _____ Do a primary survey of the victim.

   _____ Do a secondary survey of the victim.

Answers

1. It is important to follow the same basic steps in every emergency situation so that you don't forget anything that might affect **personal safety** (yours and the victim's) and the victim's **survival.**

2. Emergency action principles—correct order:
   3. Phone the EMS system for help.
   1. Survey the scene.
   2. Do a primary survey of the victim.
   4. Do a secondary survey of the victim.

Survey the Scene

When you hear a call for help, there are certain things that you should do. As you approach the victim, take in the whole picture. Don't look only at the victim. Take a look all around the victim. This should take only a few seconds and should not delay your caring for the victim. Here are the things you should be looking for.

Is the Scene Safe?

Is the area safe enough for you to approach the victim? For example, is there an exposed electrical wire? Are there harmful fumes? Is there danger from traffic? Once you reach the victim, decide if it is safe for you and the victim to stay where you are. Unless you or the victim is in immediate danger from a hazard at the scene, **don't move the victim.**

What Happened?

What actually happened? Look around for clues that could tell you the type of injuries the victim might have. The scene itself often gives the answers *(Fig. 3)*. If a person is lying next to a ladder, you would suspect that he or she fell off the ladder and may have broken bones. An electrical wire on the ground next to the victim might mean that the victim had an electric shock. This information is important, especially when the victim is unconscious and cannot tell you what is wrong, and there are no bystanders to give you information.

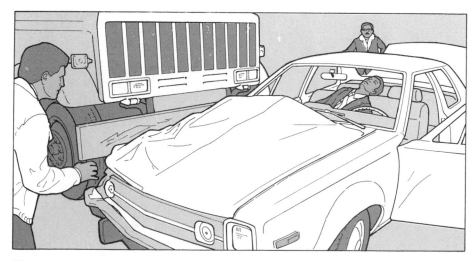

Figure 3
Survey the Scene

How Many People Are Injured?

Look beyond the victim you see at first glance. There may be other victims. One person may be screaming in pain while another, more seriously injured, may go unnoticed because he or she is unconscious. In an auto accident, car doors that are open can mean there are more victims nearby who were thrown out of or walked from the car.

Are There Bystanders Who Can Help?

If there are bystanders, use them to help you find out what happened. Maybe someone saw the victim fall. If a bystander knows the victim, ask if the victim has any medical problems. This information can help you figure out what is wrong with the victim. Bystanders can also be used to call for help and to control traffic.

Identify Yourself as a Trained Rescuer

Tell the victim and bystanders who you are and that you are trained in first aid. This may help to reassure the victim. It also may help you take charge of the situation and let someone already caring for the victim know that a trained person is on hand.

Before giving first aid to a person who is conscious, it is important that you ask permission to help the person. Legally, the person must give consent to your offer to help. In the case of an unconscious victim, consent is implied. That means that the law assumes that an unconscious victim would have given consent if conscious.

Review Questions

Fill in the blanks with the right word(s) and check the best answer.

3. Complete the four questions that you should ask yourself when you first survey the scene in an emergency.

   1. Is the area_____for you and the victim?

   2. What actually_____to the victim?

   3. How many people are_____?

   4. Are there any_____who can help?

4. Why should you identify yourself as a rescuer trained in first aid to the victim and bystanders? (Check **two**.)
   ☐ a. To reassure the victim.
   ☐ b. So that someone already caring for the victim will know you are trained in first aid.
   ☐ c. To learn the names of witnesses.

Answers

3. 1. Is the area **safe** for you and the victim?
2. What actually **happened** to the victim?
3. How many people are **injured?**
4. Are there any **bystanders** who can help?

4. You should identify yourself as a rescuer trained in first aid to the victim and bystanders:
a. **to reassure the victim,** and
b. **so that someone already caring for the victim will know you are trained in first aid.**

Once you reach the injured person, you must find out what's wrong. The victim can be a source of information, but may not know all that is wrong, or may not know that he or she is seriously injured. This can occur when the victim's thoughts are occupied with other things, such as the welfare of others. It may be clear that an arm or leg is broken, or that there is bleeding, but there may be a more serious injury that isn't so obvious. The pain of one injury may hide another.

No matter what the emergency, you should follow the same basic steps in finding out what's wrong with the victim. First, you will do a primary survey. Next, you will phone the EMS system for help. Then you will do a secondary survey.

Do a Primary Survey

The primary survey is a series of checks to find conditions that are an immediate threat to the victim's life. When you do a primary survey, you are checking the condition of the body's two most vital systems—the respiratory system and the circulatory system.

This is done by checking the **ABCs:**

Airway: Does the person have an open airway (air passage that allows the victim to breathe)?

Breathing: Is the person breathing?

Circulation: Is the person's heart beating? (Does the person have a pulse?)
Is the person bleeding severely?

You will find out how to open an airway and check for breathing and circulation in Chapter 3. If you find a problem with the person's airway, breathing, or circulation during the primary survey, then you must take care of it right away. (Note: Control of bleeding is taught in other American Red Cross first aid courses.)

Review Questions

Check the best answer and fill in the blanks with the right word(s).

5. The purpose of the primary survey is to:
   ☐ a. Find conditions that are an immediate threat to life.
   ☐ b. Find out if the person has any broken bones.

6. When you are doing the primary survey, you should check the person's **ABCs:**

   A._____

   B._____

   C._____

Answers

5. a. The purpose of the primary survey is to **find conditions that are an immediate threat to life.**

6. When you are doing a primary survey, you should check the person's **ABCs:**
   A. **Airway**
   B. **Breathing**
   C. **Circulation** (check for **pulse** and severe **bleeding**)

Phone the Emergency Medical Services (EMS) System for Help

Depending on the situation, either you or a bystander should make the telephone call for help. Since you will have had training in dealing with emergencies, it will usually be best for you to stay with the victim and let a bystander phone the EMS system for help *(Fig. 4)*. When you instruct someone to call the EMS system, you should do the following:

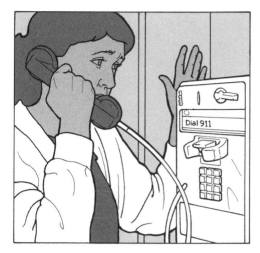

Figure 4
Phone the EMS System

1. Send two or more bystanders to make the call, if possible. This will make it more likely that the call is made.

2. Give the caller(s) the EMS telephone number to call. (In some communities, this is 911.) Dial "0" (the operator) only if you do not know the special EMS number. (Emergency telephone numbers sometimes are printed on the inside front cover of telephone directories and on pay phones.)

3. Tell the caller(s) to give the following important information to the dispatcher:
   - **Where** the emergency is. Give the exact address or location and the name of the city or town. It is helpful to give nearby intersections, landmarks, the name of the building, the floor, and the room number.
   - **Telephone number from which the call is being made.**
   - **Caller's name.**
   - **What happened:** heart attack, cardiac arrest, car accident, house on fire, etc.
   - **How many persons injured.**
   - **Condition of victim(s).**
   - **Help (first aid) being given.**

The caller(s) should not hang up until the dispatcher hangs up. It is important to make sure that the dispatcher has all the information needed to get the right help to the scene quickly.

4. Instruct the caller(s) to report back to you after making the call and to tell you what the dispatcher said.

Do a Secondary Survey

The secondary survey of a victim is a series of checks for injuries or other problems that are not an immediate threat to life, but which could cause problems if not corrected. For example, during the secondary survey, the rescuer may find that the person has a broken bone. This may not be immediately life threatening, but could become a serious problem if ignored.

The secondary survey has three parts:
1. Interviewing the victim.
2. Determining if breathing, pulse, and body temperature are normal.
3. Checking the person from head to toe, looking for injuries.

Most of the emergencies that you will learn about in this course are discovered during the primary survey. For this reason the secondary survey is not covered in great detail in this course. For a conscious heart attack victim, however, you will need to interview the person as part of the secondary survey after you have sent someone to phone the EMS system for help. (All three parts of the secondary survey are covered in greater detail in other American Red Cross courses.)

Interview the Victim

During the interview, talk to the victim to find out as much as you can. Try to get his or her name and age; find out what happened. Does the person have any medical problems that might have led to this emergency?

Ask if there is any pain, where it hurts, and how long it has hurt. This information is important to EMS and hospital emergency department personnel who will continue caring for the victim. It is important that you interview the victim and get this information as soon as possible, because he or she may lose consciousness. Writing the information down is a good way to make sure you will give it to EMS personnel accurately.

Review Questions

Check the best answer and fill in the blanks with the right word(s).

7. What is the chief purpose of the secondary survey?
   □ a. To look for injuries or other problems that are not an immediate threat to life, but that could be dangerous if not corrected.
   □ b. To find out the victim's medical history.
   □ c. To find out where the victim lives.

8. What should you tell the dispatcher when you phone for help?
   1. _____ the emergency is.
   2. _____ _____ from which the call is being made.
   3. Your _____.
   4. What _____.
   5. How many _____.
   6. _____ of victim(s).
   7. _____ being given.

9. Why is it important to interview a conscious heart attack victim?
   □ a. To be able to contact the victim's family and inform them fully about the victim's condition.
   □ b. To get accurate information about the victim to give to EMS and emergency department personnel who will be caring for the victim.

Answers

7. a. The chief purpose of the secondary survey is **to look for injuries or other problems that are not an immediate threat to life, but that could be dangerous if not corrected.**

8. What should you tell the EMS dispatcher when you phone for help?
   1. **Where** the emergency is.
   2. **Telephone number** from which the call is being made.
   3. Your **name.**
   4. What **happened.**
   5. How many **injured.**
   6. **Condition** of victim(s).
   7. **Help** (first aid) being given.

9. b. It is important to interview a conscious heart attack victim **to get accurate information about the victim to give to EMS and emergency department personnel who will be caring for the victim.**

Summary of Emergency Action Principles

Remember, follow these steps for all victims:
1. Survey the scene.
2. Do a primary survey.
3. Phone the EMS system for help.
4. Do a secondary survey.

If you find a problem during the primary survey, you will have to deal with it immediately. For example, if the victim's heart has stopped, you should begin CPR and have someone phone the EMS system for help. In this case, you would not do a secondary survey. On the other hand, if you find no life-threatening problems during the primary survey, you would go on to the secondary survey. For example, if the person is having a heart attack and is conscious you should call the EMS system for help and begin the secondary survey by interviewing the victim.

3 What to Do When Breathing Stops (Rescue Breathing)

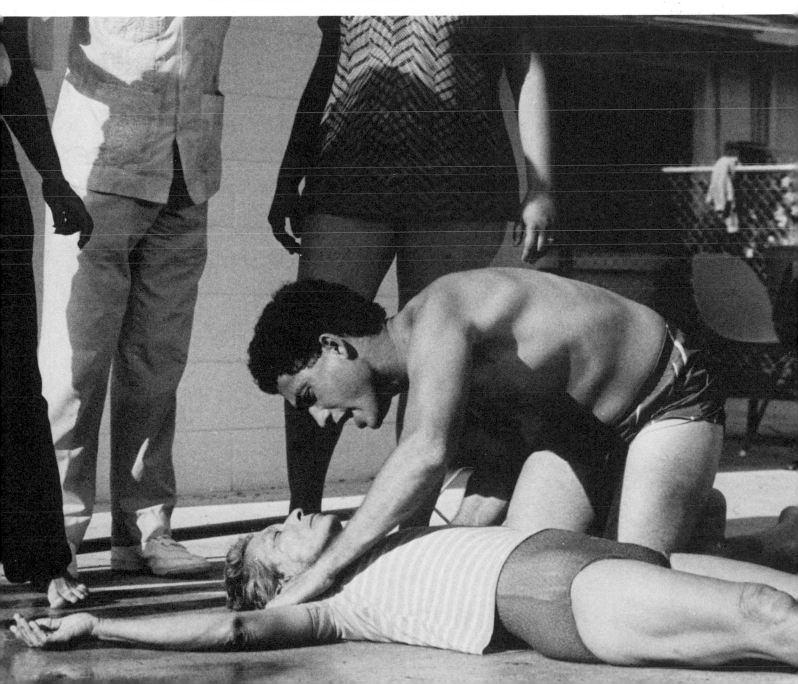

What to Do When Breathing Stops
(Rescue Breathing)

In this chapter, you will learn how to perform **artificial respiration,** also called **rescue breathing.** The primary survey will tell you if you need to give rescue breathing. Rescue breathing is given to someone whose breathing has stopped, but whose heart is still beating.

You will also learn how respiratory emergencies happen, the purpose of rescue breathing, and why it works. You will practice checking the **ABCs** (**A**irway, **B**reathing, **C**irculation) as part of the primary survey, and you will also practice rescue breathing. You will practice some of these skills on each other and some on a manikin.

Objectives

By the time you finish reading this chapter, you should be able to do the following:

1. Describe how the respiratory and circulatory systems work to provide the body's cells with oxygen.
2. Describe the purpose of rescue breathing and how rescue breathing works.
3. Give one example of each of the two types of airway obstruction.
4. Describe when rescue breathing is needed.
5. Describe how to position a person for rescue breathing.
6. Describe how to give rescue breathing.

Staying Alive

Your body is built from many millions of cells. To stay alive, these cells need a constant supply of oxygen. Right this minute, the vital flow of oxygen to your cells is being provided by two important body systems working together: the **respiratory system** and the **circulatory system.**

The **respiratory system** brings the oxygen needed to keep us alive into the body. Oxygen is part of the air we breathe. When we breathe in, air enters the body through the nose and mouth. It travels down the throat, through the windpipe, and into the lungs. The pathway from the nose and mouth to the lungs is called the **airway.** In order for air to enter the lungs, the airway must be open. In the lungs, the oxygen in the air is picked up by the blood and carried to all the cells of the body through the **circulatory system.**

If either the respiratory or circulatory system stops working or becomes damaged, then the supply of oxygen to the cells is decreased and the person may soon die. In cases like this, the victim needs rescue breathing or CPR to stay alive until advanced medical help arrives.

Respiratory Emergencies

A **respiratory emergency** occurs when a person's normal breathing stops or when breathing is so reduced that the person can't breathe enough air to stay alive. Without a constant supply of oxygen the brain will begin to die within four to six minutes. In such cases, rescue breathing is needed immediately if the person is to live. Rescue breathing is a way of breathing air into someone's lungs when natural breathing has stopped or a person can't breathe properly on his or her own.

Rescue breathing works because the air you breathe into the victim contains more than enough oxygen to keep that person alive. The air you take in with every breath contains about 21 percent oxygen, but your body uses only a small part of that. The air you breathe out of your own lungs and into the lungs of the victim contains about 16 percent oxygen. That is enough oxygen to keep someone alive.

What to Do When Breathing Stops (Rescue Breathing)

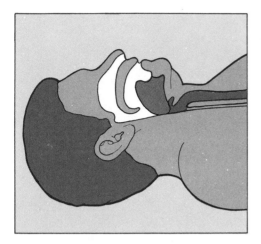

Figure 5
Tongue Obstructing Airway

Causes of Respiratory Emergencies

Respiratory emergencies most commonly happen when the airway becomes obstructed in some way. There are two types of airway obstruction: **anatomic obstruction** and **mechanical obstruction.**

Anatomic obstruction occurs when the tongue or tissues of the throat block a person's airway. This can happen in two ways:

- The airway can be blocked by the back of the tongue dropping down into the throat. This is the most common cause of airway obstruction and often occurs when an unconscious person is lying on his or her back *(Fig. 5)*.
- A person's airway also can be blocked when tissues in the throat swell. Swelling can be caused by injuries such as a blow to the neck, or by burns, allergies, insect stings and bites, poisons, and certain diseases and illnesses.

Mechanical obstruction occurs when the airway is partly or completely blocked by:

- A solid object, such as a piece of food or a small toy.
- Fluids, including vomit, blood, mucus, or saliva.

There are several other and less common causes of respiratory failure. Among them are electrocution, drowning, shock, breathing toxic substances, injury to the chest or lungs, and the effects of certain drugs.

Review Questions

Fill in the blanks with the right word(s) and check the best answer.

1. You give rescue breathing when a person has stopped

   _____.

2. Rescue breathing works because the _____ you breathe out of your own lungs and into the lungs of the victim contains enough _____ to keep the person alive until medical help arrives.

3. A person's airway can become obstructed if:

   a. The back of the _____ drops into the throat.

   b. The tissues in the _____ swell.

   c. A _____ _____ gets stuck in the airway.

   d. _____ collect in the airway.

4. The most common cause of airway obstruction in an unconscious person is:

   ☐ a. The back of the tongue blocking the throat.

   ☐ b. An object blocking the airway.

   ☐ c. Fluids blocking the airway.

Answers

1. You give rescue breathing when a person has stopped **breathing.**

2. Rescue breathing works because the **air** you breathe out of your own lungs into the lungs of the victim contains enough **oxygen** to keep the person alive until medical help arrives.

3. A person's airway can become obstructed if:
   a. The back of the **tongue** drops into the throat.
   b. The tissues in the **throat** swell.
   c. A **solid object** gets stuck in the airway.
   d. **Fluids** collect in the airway.

4. a. The most common cause of airway obstruction in an unconscious person is **the back of the tongue blocking the throat.**

Rescue Breathing

If you find someone collapsed on the floor, here's what you should do. Quickly survey the scene and begin doing a primary survey.

1. **Check for Unresponsiveness**
   The first thing you should do is check to see if the person is conscious. Kneel down beside the person, tap or gently shake the person, and shout, "Are you OK?" *(Fig. 6)*.

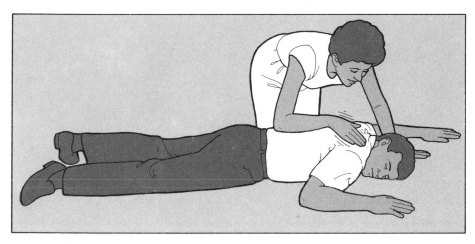

Figure 6
Check for Unresponsiveness

2. Shout for Help

If the person does not move or answer, shout for help *(Fig. 7)*. You do this to get the attention of people you can ask to phone the EMS system for help after you have completed the primary survey.

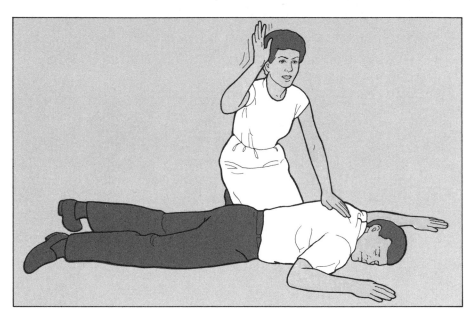

Figure 7
Shout for Help

3. Position the Victim

Move the victim onto his or her back. To do this, roll the victim as a unit, as shown in *Fig. 8*. This will help to avoid twisting the body and making any other injuries worse.

- Kneel facing the victim, midway between the victim's hips and shoulders.
- Straighten the victim's legs if necessary.
- Move the arm closest to you so that it is stretched out above the victim's head.
- Lean over the victim and place one hand on the victim's shoulder and the other on the victim's hip.

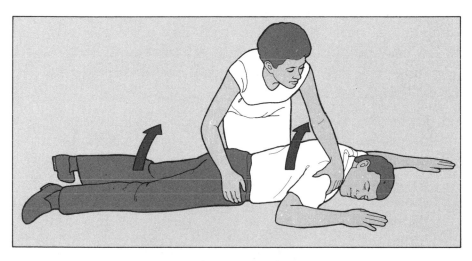

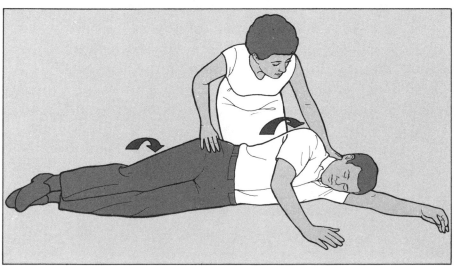

Figure 8
Position the Victim

- Roll the victim toward you as a single unit by pulling slowly and evenly.
- As you roll the victim onto his or her back, move your hand from the shoulder to support the back of the head and neck during the roll.
- Place the victim's arm nearest you alongside the victim's body.

It is important to position the victim on the back as quickly as possible. It should take no more than 10 seconds to do this.

Note: Most conditions requiring rescue breathing or CPR are not due to or associated with major injuries. However, a small number of the victims who require rescue breathing or CPR may have received a serious injury to the head, neck, or back. Moving these victims, or opening the airway as described below, may result in further injury. Additional methods for handling these victims are discussed in the American Red Cross: Basic Life Support course.

4. **Open the Airway**

   Immediately open the victim's airway. This is the most important action for successful resuscitation. The technique for opening the airway is called the **head-tilt/ chin-lift.** The head-tilt/chin-lift lifts the tongue away from the back of the throat and opens the airway. It is done by tilting the person's head back and, at the same time, lifting up on the chin *(Fig. 9)*.

   - Place your hand which is closest to the victim's head on the victim's forehead and apply firm backward pressure with the palm of your hand to tilt the head back.
   - Place the fingers of your other hand under the bony part of the victim's lower jaw near the chin and lift to bring the chin forward.
   - Lift the jaw until the teeth are nearly brought together. Do not close the victim's mouth. You can use your thumb to help keep the mouth open. Do not press on the soft tissue under the chin. This might close the airway.

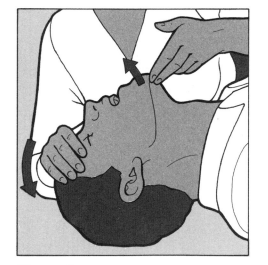

Figure 9
Head-tilt/Chin-lift

5. Check for Breathlessness (Look, listen, and feel for breathing.)

With the head tilted back and the chin lifted, check to see if the victim is breathing *(Fig. 10)*. Tilting the head back opens the airway and may in itself restore breathing *(Fig. 11)*. To check breathing:

- Keep the victim's head tilted back and the chin lifted in order to keep the airway open.
- Place your ear just above the victim's mouth and nose and look at the victim's chest.
- "Look, listen, and feel." **Look** for the chest to rise and fall, **listen** for breathing, and **feel** for air coming out of the victim's nose and mouth. Do this for three to five seconds.

If the victim is breathing, you will see chest movement and hear and feel escaping air at your ear and cheek. Chest movement alone does not mean that the victim is breathing.

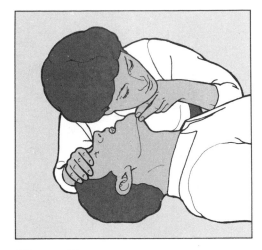

Figure 10
Check for Breathlessness

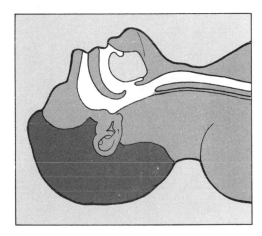

Figure 11
Open Airway

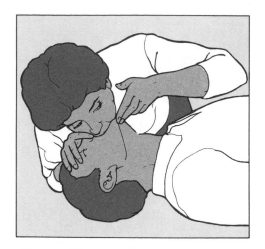

Figure 12
Mouth-to-Mouth Breathing

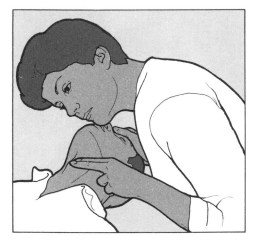

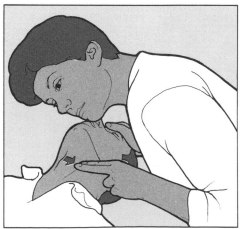

Figure 13
Locate and Feel Carotid Pulse

6. Give Two Full Breaths

If the victim is not breathing, you must get air into his or her lungs at once *(Fig. 12)*.

- While keeping the airway open with the head-tilt/chin-lift, gently pinch the victim's nose shut with the thumb and index finger of the hand that is maintaining backward pressure on the forehead.
- Open your mouth wide. Take a deep breath. Seal your lips tightly around the outside of the victim's mouth.
- Give two full breaths at the rate of 1 to 1½ seconds per breath. Pause between breaths just long enough for you to take another breath. Watch for the chest to rise while you breathe into the victim and for the chest to fall after you remove your mouth from the victim. Listen and feel for air escaping as the victim's chest falls.

If you feel resistance when you breathe into the victim, and air will not go in, the most likely cause is that you may not have tilted the head back far enough and the tongue may be blocking the airway. Retilt the head and give two full breaths.

If air still does not go into the victim's lungs, the victim's airway may be blocked by food or some other material. You will learn how to deal with obstructions caused by food and other objects in Chapter 4, "What to Do for Choking."

7. Check for a Pulse at the Side of the Neck

Check to see if the victim's heart is beating by feeling for a pulse at the side of the neck. This pulse is called the **carotid pulse** *(Fig. 13)*.

- While keeping the victim's head tilted back with one hand on the forehead, use your other hand to find the pulse. First, place your index and middle fingers on the Adam's apple. (Men and women both have Adam's apples.)

  Then slide your fingers toward you into the groove between the windpipe and the muscle at the side of the neck. This is where the carotid pulse is located.

- Press gently with your fingertips to feel for the beat of the pulse. Be sure to feel for the pulse on the side of the neck closest to you. **Do not use your thumb** (because you may feel your own pulse).

  Feel for the carotid pulse for at least 5 seconds, but no more than 10 seconds.

8. Phone the EMS System

After you have checked the pulse, you will have enough information about the victim's condition to give to the bystanders you are sending to phone the EMS system. In Chapter 2, you learned what to tell bystanders when calling the EMS system. Now you can add the last important piece of information: details of the victim's condition. Tell them whether the victim is conscious, breathing, and has a pulse.

9. Begin Rescue Breathing

If you feel a pulse and the victim is not breathing, then you must begin rescue breathing. (If you do not feel a pulse, the victim's heart has stopped and you must start CPR, which you will learn later.)

- Keep the airway open.

- Give one breath every five seconds at the rate of 1 to 1½ seconds per breath, watching for the chest to rise. A good way to do this is to count, "One one-thousand, two one-thousand, three one-thousand, four one-thousand, b-r-e-a-t-h-e," and then give a breath.

- Between breaths, remove your mouth from the victim and look for the chest to fall as you listen and feel at the victim's mouth and nose for the air to come out. You should also listen for the return of breathing.

10. Recheck Pulse

After one minute (about 12 breaths), you should check the victim's pulse.

- Keep the airway open and feel for the carotid pulse for five seconds.

  If there is a pulse, then check for breathing for three to five seconds. If breathing is present, keep the airway open and monitor breathing and pulse closely. This means that you should look, listen, and feel for breathing while you keep checking the pulse. If there is no breathing, continue rescue breathing and keep checking the pulse every minute.

Continue to give rescue breathing until:

- The victim begins breathing on his or her own.
- Another trained rescuer takes over for you.
- Emergency medical services personnel arrive and take over.
- You are too exhausted to continue.

Review Questions

Fill in the blanks with the right word(s) and check the best answer.

5. You see someone collapse on the sidewalk in front of you. You survey the scene and decide it is safe. What should you do upon reaching the victim?

Check for _____ and open the

_____.

6. How do you open the airway?
- ☐ a. Tilt the head and lift the chin.
- ☐ b. Blow into the victim's nose.
- ☐ c. Push down on the chin.

7. How often should you give rescue breaths?
- ☐ a. Give one breath every second.
- ☐ b. Give one breath every five seconds.
- ☐ c. Give one breath every 30 seconds.

8. You should continue rescue breathing until one of four things happens. These four things are:

a. The victim starts _____.

b. _____ _____ arrive and take over.

c. Another trained rescuer _____ _____ for you.

d. You are too _____ to continue.

Answers

5. The first thing you do if you find a person collapsed is to check for **unresponsiveness** and open the **airway**.

6. a. To open the airway, **tilt the head and lift the chin.**

7. b. **Give one rescue breath every five seconds.**

8. You should continue rescue breathing until one of the following happens.
a. The victim starts **breathing.**
b. **EMS personnel** arrive and take over.
c. Another trained rescuer **takes over** for you.
d. You are too **exhausted** to continue.

Introduction

This course has three practice sessions. In these practice sessions you will learn how to perform rescue breathing, how to help someone who is choking, and how to perform CPR (cardiopulmonary resuscitation).

During each practice session you will use a skill sheet to guide you through the skills you will learn. On the page before each skill sheet are the directions for that practice session. Please read the directions carefully. As you read through the checklists on the skill sheets, you will see that each skill is made up of a number of steps.

You will practice each skill in groups of two or three. One person will be the rescuer and will perform the skills on the skill sheet. The second person will read the directions on the skill sheet to the rescuer. If there are three people in your group and you are practicing on a manikin, the third person will observe the rescuer perform the skills and will check the rescuer's performance. For some skills, you will practice on one another and not on a manikin. When this happens, the third person will be the victim.

Partner Check

When you first start practicing, have a partner read the skill sheet checklist aloud to you. It is important that your partner reads **all** the steps on the checklist to you. The checklists not only help you learn the steps in the correct order, but also give you information about the victim's condition.

You should practice until you can perform the skills correctly and confidently, and in the right order, without having your partner read the directions to you.

When you can do the skills correctly without coaching from your partner, your partner should watch you go through the whole procedure and check off each step in the "Partner Check" column on the skill sheet as you do it.

At the end of each skill sheet is a section called "What to Do Next." Your partner will read this section to you only after you feel comfortable that you know the skill. This section will give you practice in deciding how to change the care you are giving in response to changes in the victim's condition. Your partner will prompt you by giving you information about the victim's condition, and you will make a decision about what to do next.

After your partner has checked you, change places with your partner and go through the same procedure while he or she practices the skills.

If you need help during the practice session, ask your instructor or reread the appropriate section in this workbook.

Instructor Skill Test

When all the members of your group are ready to be tested, ask the instructor to test your skills.

During the skill test, the instructor will ask you to go through the whole procedure without prompting. If the instructor sees a serious error, he or she will stop testing and correct you. You will be asked to practice some more before being tested again. Ask a partner to work with you. When you have practiced and feel that you are ready to be tested again, ask the instructor to retest you. When you have completed the procedure correctly, the instructor will sign your workbook.

Practice on Each Other

As stated above, you will practice some skills on a partner. By practicing on each other, you will learn how it feels to work on a real person. For example, you will learn what a real carotid pulse feels like.

When practicing on a partner, follow the checklist directions but do not make mouth-to-mouth contact; do not give actual rescue breaths; do not perform chest compressions; and do not perform abdominal thrusts or chest thrusts.

Practice on a Manikin

Before you start working on the manikin, clean the face and the inside of the mouth with disinfecting solution according to the directions given on the inside front cover of this book. Be sure that the manikin's face and mouth have been cleaned with disinfecting solution before each new member of your group practices, and whenever you change places and begin practicing on the manikin.

Health Precautions

Before you start practicing, read "Some Health Precautions and Guidelines" at the front of your workbook. If you have any questions or if there is any reason that you should not take part in the practice sessions, it is important that you talk with your instructor.

Practice Session: Rescue Breathing (Adult)

The Rescue Breathing practice session is the first of the three practice sessions. During this practice session, you will first practice on a partner. If possible, a third person should read the skill checklist as you practice.

Remember: **When you practice on a partner, do not make mouth-to-mouth contact or give actual rescue breaths.**

When you practice on a manikin, you will practice all the steps and will give actual breaths.

Make sure that the manikin's face and mouth are cleaned with disinfecting solution before each person starts practicing on the manikin.

Before you start practicing, carefully read the skill sheet checklist on pages 51 through 54 in this workbook.

If you don't remember how to use the checklist, read pages 47 and 48 in your workbook.

Skill Sheet

You find a person lying on the ground, not moving. You should survey the scene to see if it is safe, and to get some idea of what happened. Then begin doing a primary survey by checking the ABCs.

Remember: When using a real person as a victim, **do not make mouth-to-mouth contact or give actual rescue breaths.**

Partner Check
Instructor Check

☐ ☐ **Check for Unresponsiveness**

Tap or gently shake victim

Rescuer shouts "Are you OK?"

Partner/Instructor says "Unconscious"

Rescuer says "Unconscious"

Rescuer shouts "Help!"

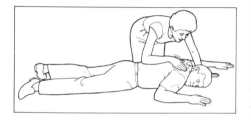

☐ ☐ **Position the Victim**

– Roll victim onto back, if necessary

Kneel facing victim, midway between victim's hips and shoulders

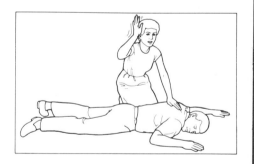

Straighten victim's legs, if necessary, and move arm closest to you above victim's head

Lean over victim, and place one hand on victim's shoulder and other hand on victim's hip

Roll victim toward you as a single unit; as you roll victim, move your hand from shoulder to support back of head and neck

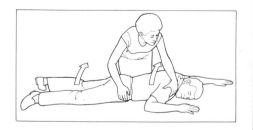

Place victim's arm nearest you alongside victim's body

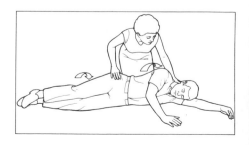

Partner Check
Instructor Check

☐ ☐ **Open the Airway:** Use head-tilt/chin-lift method

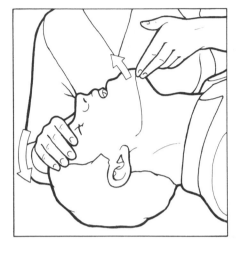

Place one hand on victim's forehead

– Place fingers of other hand under bony part of lower jaw near chin

– Tilt head and lift jaw—avoid closing victim's mouth

☐ ☐ **Check for Breathlessness**

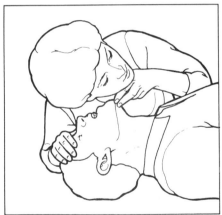

– Maintain open airway

– Place your ear over victim's mouth and nose

– Look at chest, listen and feel for breathing for 3 to 5 seconds

Partner/Instructor says "No breathing"

Rescuer repeats "No breathing"

☐ ☐ **Give 2 Full Breaths**

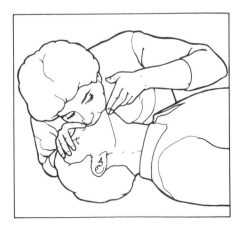

– Maintain open airway

– Pinch nose shut

– Open your mouth wide, take a deep breath, and make a tight seal around outside of victim's mouth

– Give 2 full breaths at the rate of 1 to 1½ seconds per breath

– Observe chest rise and fall; listen and feel for escaping air

☐ ☐ **Check for Pulse**

– Maintain head tilt with one hand on forehead

– Locate Adam's apple with middle and index fingers of hand closest to victim's feet

– Slide fingers down into groove of neck on side closest to you

– Feel for carotid pulse for 5 to 10 seconds

Partner/Instructor says "No breathing, but there is a pulse"

Rescuer repeats "No breathing, but there is a pulse"

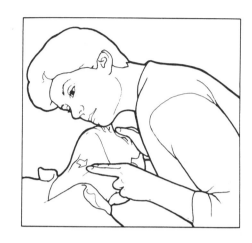

☐ ☐ **Phone the EMS System for Help**

– Tell someone to call for an ambulance

Rescuer says "No breathing, has a pulse, call _____." (Local emergency number or Operator)

☐ ☐ **Now Begin Rescue Breathing**

– Maintain open airway

– Pinch nose shut

– Open your mouth wide, take a deep breath, and make a tight seal around outside of victim's mouth

– Give 1 breath every 5 seconds at the rate of 1 to 1½ seconds per breath

– Observe chest rise and fall; listen and feel for escaping air and the return of breathing

Continue for 1 minute—about 12 breaths

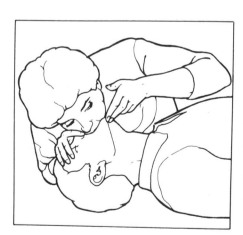

Practice Session: Rescue Breathing (Adult)

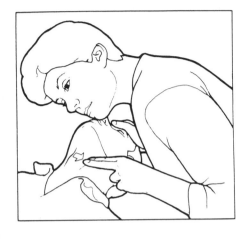

Partner Check
Instructor Check

☐ ☐ **Recheck Pulse**

– Tilt head

– Locate carotid pulse and feel for 5 seconds

Partner/Instructor says "Has pulse"

Rescuer repeats "Has pulse"

– Next look, listen, and feel for breathing for 3 to 5 seconds

Partner/Instructor says "No breathing"

Rescuer repeats "No breathing"

☐ ☐ **Continue Rescue Breathing**

– Maintain open airway

– Give 1 breath every 5 seconds at the rate of 1 to 1½ seconds per breath

– Recheck pulse every minute

☐ ☐ **What to Do Next**

While the rescuer is rechecking pulse and breathing, the partner should read one of the following statements:

1. Victim is breathing but is still unconscious.

2. Victim has a pulse but is not breathing.

Based on this information, the rescuer should make a decision about what to do next, and continue giving the right care.

Final Instructor Check_____

More About Rescue Breathing

Air in the Stomach

Sometimes during rescue breathing the rescuer may breathe air into the victim's stomach. Air in the stomach can be a serious problem. It can cause the victim to vomit. When an unconscious person vomits, the stomach contents may go into the lungs. That can lead to death.

Air can enter the stomach in three ways:
- When the rescuer keeps breathing into the victim after the chest has risen. This causes extra air to fill the stomach.
- When the rescuer has not tilted the victim's head back far enough to open the airway completely and must breathe at greater pressure to fill the victim's lungs.
- When the rescue breaths are given too quickly. Quick breaths are given with higher pressure, which causes air to enter the stomach.

To avoid forcing air into the stomach, make sure you keep the victim's head tilted all the way back. Breathe into the victim only enough to make the chest rise. Don't give breaths too quickly; pause between breaths long enough to let the victim's lungs empty and for you to get another breath.

If you notice that the victim's stomach has begun to bulge, make sure that the head is tilted back far enough and make sure you are not breathing into the victim too hard or too fast.

Vomiting

Sometimes while you are helping an unconscious victim, the victim may vomit. If this happens, turn the victim's head and body to the side, quickly wipe the material out of the victim's mouth, and continue where you left off.

Mouth-to-Nose Breathing

There are a few situations when you may not be able to make a good enough seal over a person's mouth to perform rescue breathing. For example, the person's jaw or mouth may be injured during an accident, or the jaw may be shut too tight to open, or your mouth may be too small. In such cases, **mouth-to-nose breathing** should be done as follows:

- Maintain the backward head-tilt position with one hand on the forehead. Use the other hand to close the mouth **(Fig. 14)**, making sure to push on the chin and not on the throat.
- Open your mouth wide, take a deep breath, seal your mouth tightly around the person's nose, and breathe full breaths into the person's nose **(Fig. 15)**, as described above for the mouth-to-mouth method. Open the person's mouth between breaths if possible to allow air to come out **(Fig. 16)**.

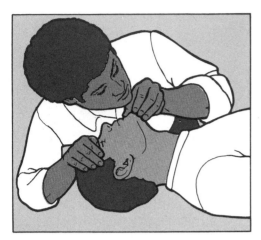

Figure 14
Close Mouth for Mouth-to-Nose Breathing

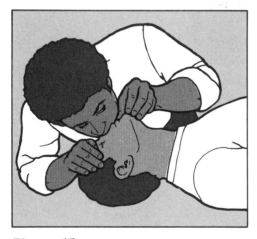

Figure 15
Mouth-to-Nose Breathing

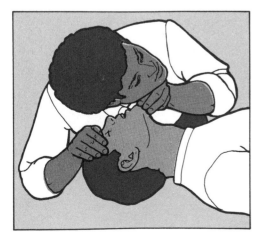

Figure 16
Check for Air Coming Out

Mouth-to-Stoma Breathing

There are some people who have had surgery to remove all or part of the upper end of their windpipe. They breathe through an opening called a **stoma** in the front of the neck *(Fig. 17)*. This takes the air right into the windpipe, bypassing both the mouth and nose.

Most people with this condition wear a bracelet or necklace or carry a card identifying their condition. In an emergency, you may not have time to search for a medical card, so it is important to look at the neck area during the primary survey to see if the person has a stoma.

To give rescue breathing to someone with a stoma, you must give breaths through the stoma and not through the mouth or nose.

In **mouth-to-stoma** breathing, you follow the same basic steps as in mouth-to-mouth breathing, except that you:

1. Look, listen, and feel for breathing with your ear held over the stoma *(Fig. 18)*.
2. Give breaths into the stoma, breathing at the same rate as for mouth-to-mouth breathing *(Fig. 19)*.

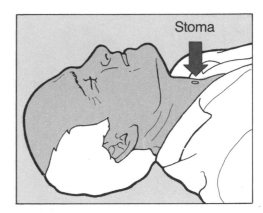

Figure 17
Victim With a Stoma

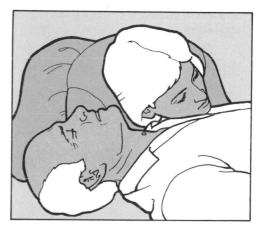

Figure 18
Check for Breathing

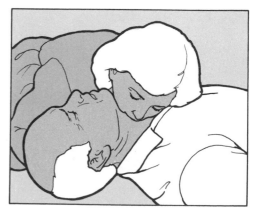

Figure 19
Mouth-to-Stoma Breathing

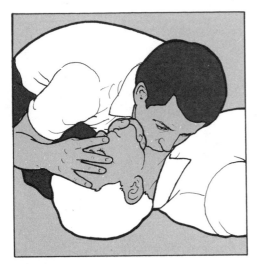

Figure 20
**Mouth-to-Stoma Breathing for
Partial Stoma**

There are several other important things you should remember when you give rescue breathing to someone who breathes through a stoma.

- Don't tilt the victim's head back.
- Don't breathe air into the victim through his or her nose or mouth. This may fill the victim's stomach with air.
- Never block the stoma, since it is the only way the victim has to breathe.
- In some instances a person who has had only part of the upper end of his or her windpipe removed may breathe through the stoma as well as the nose and mouth. If the person's chest does not rise when you breathe through the stoma, you should close off the mouth and nose ***(Fig. 20)*** and continue breathing through the stoma.

Victims With Dentures (False Teeth)

If a person who needs rescue breathing is wearing dentures, leave the dentures in place if they have not moved. They will give support to the mouth and cheeks during mouth-to-mouth breathing. Even if the dentures are loose, the head-tilt/chin-lift described earlier may help keep them in place. If the dentures become so loose that they block the airway or make it difficult for you to give breaths, take them out.

4 *What to Do for Choking*

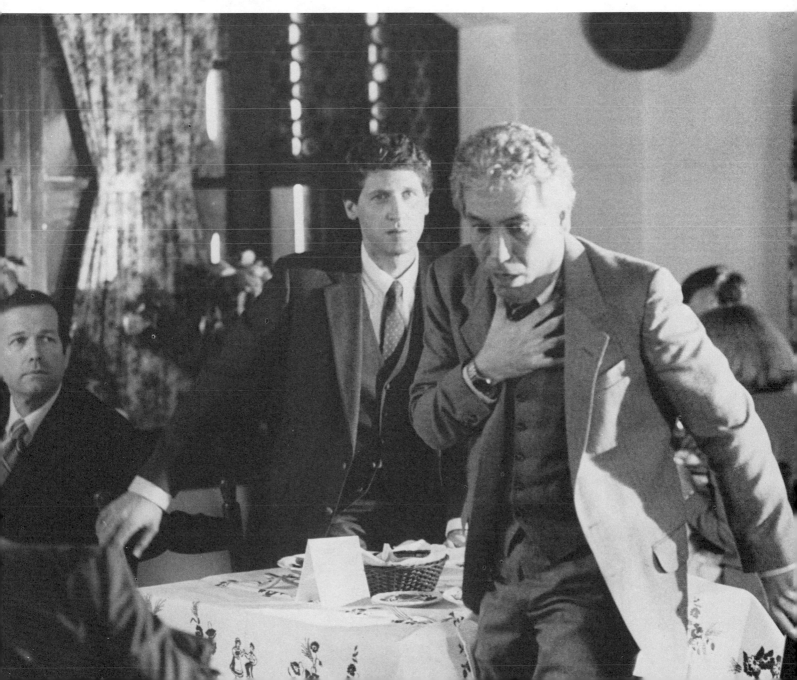

When someone's airway gets blocked by a piece of food or some other object, the person can quickly stop breathing, lose consciousness, and die. In this chapter, you will learn how to tell if a person is choking. You will learn how to tell whether the person has an airway obstruction that requires first aid, and you will learn the first aid to clear an obstructed airway.

Objectives

By the time you finish this chapter, you should be able to do the following:

1. List at least two reasons why people choke.
2. Describe the difference between airway obstructions that require first aid (complete airway obstruction or partial obstruction with poor air exchange) and those obstructions that can best be cleared by the victim's own efforts (partial airway obstruction with good air exchange).
3. Describe the first aid for a conscious victim who is choking.
4. Describe the first aid for an unconscious victim who is choking.

Causes and Signals of Choking

Causes of Choking

About 3,000 people will choke to death this year. Here are the most common things that lead to choking:

- Trying to swallow large pieces of food that are poorly chewed.
- Drinking alcohol before or during eating. Alcohol dulls the nerves that help you swallow.
- Wearing dentures (false teeth). Dentures make it difficult to sense the size of food when chewing and swallowing.
- Talking excitedly and laughing while eating, or eating too fast.
- Walking, playing, or running with objects in the mouth.

Choking is sometimes mistaken for a heart attack or other serious conditions. When this happens, the right kind of care may be delayed, or the wrong kind of care may be given, so it is important to know how to recognize when someone is choking.

Recognizing Airway Obstruction in a Conscious Victim

Being able to recognize an airway obstruction is the key to saving the victim. There are two types of obstruction that you need to know about—**partial airway obstruction** and **complete airway obstruction.** It is important to be able to recognize the difference between the two.

Partial Airway Obstruction

With partial airway obstruction, the person may have either "good air exchange" or "poor air exchange."

- Partial Airway Obstruction with Good Air Exchange. When a person has partial airway obstruction with good air exchange, he or she can cough forcefully. There also may be wheezing between breaths. **If the person is able to cough forcefully on his or her own, do not interfere with his or her attempts to cough up the object.** You should stay with the person and encourage him or her to continue coughing. If coughing persists, call the EMS system for help.

- Partial Airway Obstruction with Poor Air Exchange. When a person has partial airway obstruction with poor air exchange, he or she will have a weak, ineffective cough, and may make a high-pitched noise while breathing. The obstruction may begin with poor air exchange, or good air exchange may turn into poor air exchange. **Partial airway obstruction with poor air exchange should be dealt with as if it were complete airway obstruction.**

Complete Airway Obstruction

When there is complete obstruction of the airway, the person will not be able to speak, breathe, or cough. The person may clutch at the throat with one or both hands. This is the universal distress signal for choking *(Fig. 21)*. You must act right away to clear the airway.

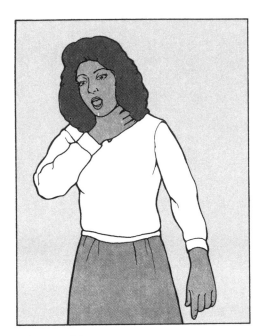

Figure 21
Universal Distress Signal for Choking

Review Questions

Fill in the blanks with the right word(s) and check the best answer.

1. These common things can lead to choking:

   a. Poorly chewed _____.

   b. Drinking _____ before and during eating.

   c. _____, which make it difficult to sense the size of food.

   d. Talking excitedly and laughing while eating, or _____ too fast.

   e. Walking, playing, or running with objects in the _____.

2. A choking victim is coughing forcefully. You should
   ☐ a. Slap the person on the back.
   ☐ b. Stay with the person and encourage him or her to continue coughing.
   ☐ c. Perform abdominal thrusts.

3. A person is coughing weakly and having great difficulty breathing. You should:
   ☐ a. Give first aid for complete airway obstruction.
   ☐ b. Let the person alone and watch him or her.

4. What is the universal distress signal for choking?
   ☐ a. Clutching at the throat.
   ☐ b. Coughing forcefully.
   ☐ c. High-pitched wheezing.

Answers

1. These common things can lead to choking:
    a. Poorly chewed **food.**
    b. Drinking **alcohol** before and during eating.
    c. **Dentures** (false teeth), which make it difficult to sense the size of food.
    d. Talking excitedly and laughing while eating, or **eating** too fast.
    e. Walking, playing, or running with objects in the **mouth.**

2. b. When a choking victim is coughing forcefully, you should **stay with the person and encourage him or her to continue coughing.**

3. a. If a person is coughing weakly and having great difficulty breathing, you should **give first aid for complete airway obstruction.**

4. a. The universal distress signal for choking is **clutching at the throat.**

First Aid for Complete Airway Obstruction (Conscious Adult)

If you see someone who looks as if he or she is choking, survey the scene as you approach the victim.

1. Begin a primary survey by asking, "Are you choking?" If the person is coughing weakly or making high-pitched noises or is not able to speak, breathe, or cough forcefully, tell the person that you are trained in first aid and offer to help.

   If there is another person nearby, have him or her phone the EMS system for help.

2. Perform abdominal thrusts (Heimlich maneuver). Abdominal thrusts may be given to a conscious victim who is standing or sitting. Stand behind the victim and wrap your arms around his or her waist. Make a fist with one hand. Place the thumb side of your fist against the middle of the victim's abdomen, just above the navel and well below the lower tip of the breastbone *(Figs. 22, 23, and 24).*

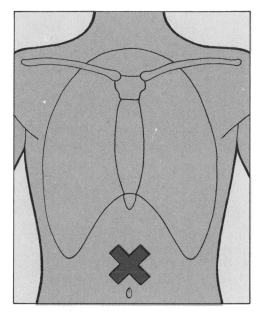

Figure 22
Location for Abdominal Thrusts

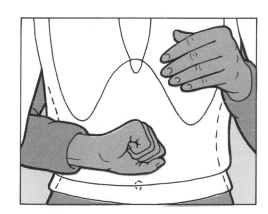

Figure 23
Hand Placement for Abdominal Thrusts

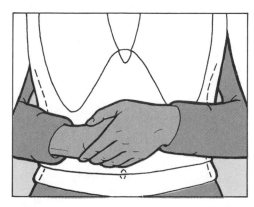

Figure 24
Location for Abdominal Thrusts

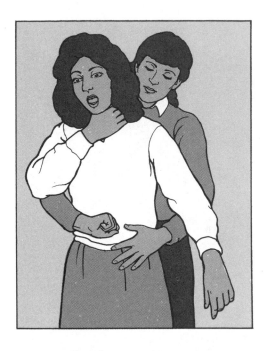

3. Grasp your fist with your other hand. Keeping your elbows out from the victim, press your fist into the person's abdomen with a quick upward thrust *(Fig. 25)*. Be sure that your fist is directly on the midline of the victim's abdomen when you press. Do not direct the thrusts to the right or to the left.

4. Repeat thrusts until the obstruction is cleared or until the person becomes unconscious. You should think of each thrust as a separate and distinct attempt to dislodge the object. (Instructions for dealing with a victim who becomes unconscious during attempts to clear the airway are presented later in this chapter as "More About First Aid for Choking.")

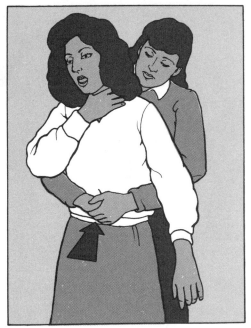

Figure 25
Giving Abdominal Thrusts

Review Questions

Check the best answer.

5. Abdominal thrusts are given to a victim who is:
   - ☐ a. Coughing weakly and making high-pitched noises.
   - ☐ b. Coughing forcefully and wheezing between breaths.

6. When you give abdominal thrusts, what part of your fist do you place against the victim?
   - ☐ a. The palm side.
   - ☐ b. The thumb side.
   - ☐ c. The knuckles.

7. When you give abdominal thrusts, where do you place your fist?
   - ☐ a. At the lower tip of the breastbone.
   - ☐ b. Just above the navel and well below the lower tip of the breastbone.
   - ☐ c. On the navel.

8. Abdominal thrusts are given:
   - ☐ a. With a quick upward thrust.
   - ☐ b. Straight back.
   - ☐ c. Inward and downward.

Answers

5. a. Abdominal thrusts are given to a victim who is **coughing weakly and making high-pitched noises.**

6. b. When you give abdominal thrusts, place **the thumb side** of your fist against the victim.

7. b. When you give abdominal thrusts, you place your fist **just above the navel and well below the lower tip of the breastbone.**

8. a. Abdominal thrusts are given **with a quick upward thrust.**

Chest Thrusts (Conscious Victim)

You may not be able to get your arms around the waist of some choking victims to deliver effective abdominal thrusts. For example, the person may be greatly overweight, or in the late stages of pregnancy. In the case of a person who is in the late stages of pregnancy, abdominal thrusts could be dangerous. In both cases, chest thrusts are performed instead. Chest thrusts are done in the following way:

1. With the person either standing or sitting, stand behind and place your arms under the person's armpits and around the chest. Place the thumb side of your fist on the middle of the breastbone. Be sure that your fist is centered right on the breastbone and not on the ribs. Also make sure that your fist is not near the lower tip of the breastbone *(Fig. 26)*.
2. Grasp your fist with your other hand and give backward thrusts *(Fig. 27)*.
3. Give thrusts until the obstruction is cleared or until the person loses consciousness. You should think of each thrust as a separate attempt to dislodge the object.

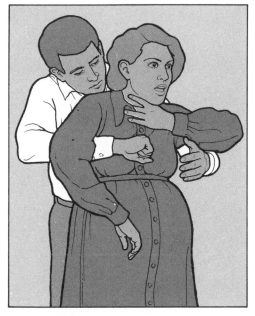

Figure 26
Hand Placement for Chest Thrusts

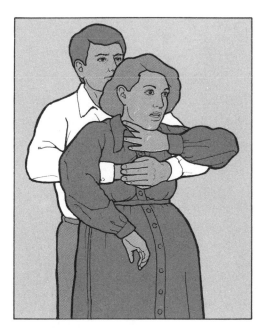

Figure 27
Giving Chest Thrusts

When to Stop

You should stop giving abdominal or chest thrusts immediately if the object is coughed up or the person begins to breathe or cough. Watch the person and make sure that the object has been removed from the airway and that the person is breathing freely again. Even after the object is coughed up, the person may have problems in breathing that are not clear to you. You should also realize that both abdominal thrusts and chest thrusts may cause internal injuries. For these reasons, the person should be taken to a hospital emergency department even if he or she seems to be breathing well.

Review Questions

Check the best answer.

9. If a choking victim is greatly overweight or in the late stages of pregnancy, which should you give?
- ☐ a. Abdominal thrusts.
- ☐ b. Chest thrusts.

10. When giving chest thrusts, place your fist:
- ☐ a. On the middle of the breastbone.
- ☐ b. On the lower end of the breastbone.
- ☐ c. On the navel.

11. You are giving chest thrusts to a woman in the late stages of pregnancy whose airway is completely blocked. Then she begins to cough forcefully. You should:
- ☐ a. Continue giving chest thrusts.
- ☐ b. Stop giving chest thrusts.

Answers

9. b. You should give **chest thrusts** if the victim is greatly overweight or in the late stages of pregnancy.

10. a. When giving chest thrusts, place your fist **on the middle of the breastbone.**

11. b. **You should stop giving chest thrusts** if the victim begins to cough forcefully.

First Aid for Complete Airway Obstruction (Unconscious Adult)

The first aid for any unconscious victim begins with a primary survey. While checking the ABCs, you may find that the victim has an obstructed airway. The procedure for identifying and giving care for an unconscious victim with a complete airway obstruction is presented below. You should start by surveying the scene and then begin a primary survey.

1. Check the victim for unresponsiveness.
2. Shout for help.
3. Position the victim on his or her back.
4. Open the airway.
5. Look, listen, and feel for breathing.
6. If the victim is not breathing, give two full breaths.
7. If you are unable to breathe air into the victim, retilt the head and give two full breaths. You may not have tilted the victim's head far enough back the first time.

If you are still unable to breathe air into the victim, tell someone to phone the EMS system for help, and do the following steps, which are described in the next few pages.

8. Give 6 to 10 abdominal thrusts.
9. Do a finger sweep to try to dislodge and remove the object from the victim's throat.
10. Open the airway and give two full breaths.

Continue these last three steps until the obstruction is cleared or EMS personnel arrive and take over.

Abdominal Thrusts

- Straddle the victim's thighs *(Fig. 28)*.

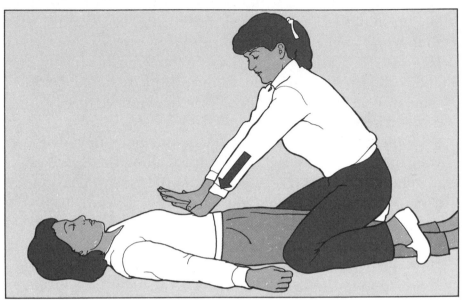

Figure 28   Abdominal Thrusts for Unconscious Victim

- Place the heel of one hand against the middle of the victim's abdomen, just above the navel and well below the lower tip of the breastbone *(Fig. 29)*. Place the other hand directly on top of the first hand with your fingers pointed toward the victim's head.
- Press into the abdomen with a quick upward thrust. Give 6 to 10 thrusts. Be sure that your hands are directly on the midline of the abdomen when you press. Do not direct the thrusts to the right or to the left. Each thrust should be a separate and distinct attempt to dislodge the object. After 6 to 10 thrusts, do a finger sweep.

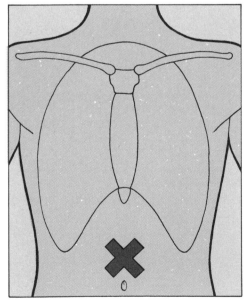

Figure 29
Location for Abdominal Thrusts

Finger Sweep

- Move from the straddle position and kneel beside the victim's head. Keeping the victim's face up, open the victim's mouth and grasp both the tongue and lower jaw between the thumb and fingers of the hand nearest the victim's legs *(Fig. 30)*. Lift the jaw. This draws the tongue away from the back of the throat and away from any object that may be lodged there. This action alone may help relieve the obstruction.
- With the jaw and tongue lifted, slide the index finger of your other hand into the mouth down along the inside of the cheek and deep into the throat to the base of the tongue *(Fig. 31)*. Then use a hooking action to dislodge the object and move it into the mouth so that it can be removed. If the object comes within reach, grasp it and remove it. Sometimes you may have to push the object against the opposite side of the throat to dislodge it and to lift it out. Be careful not to force the object deeper into the airway.

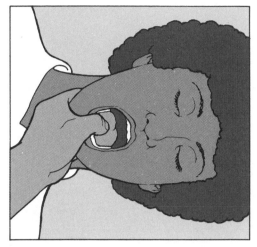

Figure 30
Grasp Tongue and Lower Jaw

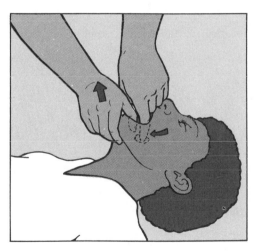

Figure 31
Finger Sweep

Review Questions

Check the best answer:

12. You encounter an unconscious victim who is not breathing. If you cannot breathe air into the victim's lungs on the first try, what should you do next?
    ☐ a. Retilt the head.
    ☐ b. Look in the mouth for an object blocking the airway.
    ☐ c. Give six to ten abdominal thrusts.

13. When you are giving abdominal thrusts to an unconscious victim, you should:
    ☐ a. Kneel beside the victim's chest.
    ☐ b. Kneel by the victim's head.
    ☐ c. Straddle the victim's thighs.

14. To give abdominal thrusts to an unconscious victim, place the heel of one hand:
    ☐ a. Over the edge of the rib cage.
    ☐ b. In the middle of the victim's abdomen slightly above the navel and well below the lower tip of the breastbone.
    ☐ c. Directly over the navel.

15. In what direction do you give abdominal thrusts to an unconscious victim?

□ a. Upward.

□ b. Straight toward the ground.

16. For an unconscious victim, how many abdominal thrusts should you give before doing a finger sweep?

□ a. 15 to 20

□ b. 6 to 10

□ c. 1 to 3

17. When doing a finger sweep, try to remove the object by:

□ a. Using a hooking action.

□ b. Poking straight into the throat.

Answers

12. a. **Retilt the head** if you cannot breathe air into the lungs of an unconscious victim who is not breathing.

13. c. **Straddle the victim's thighs** when giving abdominal thrusts to an unconscious victim.

14. b. Place the heel of one hand **in the middle of the victim's abdomen slightly above the navel and well below the lower tip of the breastbone** to give abdominal thrusts to an unconscious victim.

15. a. Give abdominal thrusts **upward.**

16. b. Give **6 to 10** abdominal thrusts before doing a finger sweep.

17. a. When doing a finger sweep, try to remove the object by **using a hooking action.**

Chest Thrusts (Unconscious Adult)

Chest thrusts should **only** be given to unconscious people who are in the late stages of pregnancy or who are greatly overweight.

You should follow the same steps as you would in giving first aid for choking to an unconscious adult, except that you substitute chest thrusts for abdominal thrusts. To give chest thrusts to an unconscious victim:

* Kneel facing the victim.
* Position your hands as you would if you were giving CPR chest compressions. (You will learn how to do this in Chapter 6, "What to Do When the Heart Stops—CPR.")
* Give 6 to 10 thrusts. Each thrust should compress the chest 1½ to 2 inches. Give slow and distinct thrusts as if you were trying to unblock the airway with each thrust.
* Do a finger sweep.
* Open the victim's airway and give two full breaths.

Repeat these last three steps until the obstruction is cleared, or EMS personnel arrive and take over.

Review

Here is the whole procedure for an unconscious victim who may be choking:

1. Check for unresponsiveness.
2. Shout for help.
3. Position the victim.
4. Open the airway.
5. Look, listen, and feel for breathing.
6. Give two full breaths.
7. Retilt the head if you are unable to breathe air into the victim.
8. Give two full breaths.

If you are still **unable** to breathe air into the victim's lungs, have someone phone the EMS system for help and:

- Give 6 to 10 abdominal thrusts (or chest thrusts if necessary).
- Do a finger sweep.
- Open the victim's airway and give two full breaths.

Continue these last three steps until the obstruction is cleared or EMS personnel arrive and take over.
If your first attempts to clear the airway are unsuccessful, **do not stop.** The longer the victim goes without oxygen, the more the muscles will relax, making it more likely that you will be able to clear the airway.

If you **are** able to breathe air into the victim's lungs, give two full breaths as you did for rescue breathing. Then check the pulse. If there is no pulse, begin CPR. If there is a pulse, and the victim is not breathing on his or her own, continue rescue breathing.

If the victim should start breathing on his or her own, monitor breathing and pulse until EMS personnel arrive and take over. This means you should maintain an open airway; look, listen, and feel for breathing; and keep checking the pulse. Keep the victim still.

Review Questions

Check the best answer.

20. You find a victim lying on the ground. You survey the scene and decide it is safe to help the victim. What should you do first?
- ☐ a. Open the airway.
- ☐ b. Attempt mouth-to-mouth breaths.
- ☐ c. Check for unresponsiveness.

21. You find an unresponsive victim. You open the victim's airway and give two full breaths, but the air will not go in. What should you do next?
- ☐ a. Retilt the head.
- ☐ b. Do a finger sweep.
- ☐ c. Give 6 to 10 abdominal thrusts.

22. You retilt the head of an unconscious victim and give two more breaths. The air still does not go in. What should you do next?
- ☐ a. Open the airway.
- ☐ b. Do a finger sweep.
- ☐ c. Give 6 to 10 abdominal thrusts.

23. After doing a finger sweep, you find that the air you breathe into the victim does go into the lungs. You can see the victim's chest rise. What should you do next?
- ☐ a. Open the airway.
- ☐ b. Check the pulse.
- ☐ c. Phone the EMS system for help.

Answers

20. c. The first thing you should do if you find a victim lying on the ground is **check for unresponsiveness.**

21. a. If you are unable to breathe air into the victim's lungs on the first try, the next thing you should do is **retilt the head.**

22. c. If you are unable to breathe air into the victim's lungs on the second try, **give 6 to 10 abdominal thrusts.**

23. b. If you are able to breathe air into the victim's lungs, the next thing you should do is **check the pulse.**

Practice Session: First Aid for Choking (Complete Airway Obstruction)

The First Aid for Choking practice session is the second of the three practice sessions. During this session you will practice on a partner, and then you will practice on a manikin. **Before you start practicing,** carefully read the following directions and the skill sheet checklist on pages 84 through 91 in this workbook.

In this practice session, you will learn two separate skills: first aid for a **conscious** adult with complete airway obstruction, and first aid for an **unconscious** adult with complete airway obstruction.

First Aid for Complete Airway Obstruction (Conscious Adult)

You will practice this skill on a partner. If possible, a third person should read the skill checklist as you practice.

Remember: **When practicing abdominal thrusts on a partner, do not give actual abdominal thrusts.**

First Aid for Complete Airway Obstruction (Unconscious Adult)

You will practice this skill on a manikin. **Do not perform finger sweeps on a manikin. Do not touch the manikin's lips or inside the mouth with your fingers.**

Skill Sheet

Remember: **When practicing abdominal thrusts on a partner, do not give actual abdominal thrusts.**

Partner Check
Instructor Check

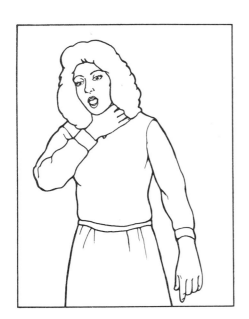

☐ ☐   **Determine If Victim Is Choking**

– Rescuer asks "Are you choking?"

Partner/Instructor says "Victim cannot cough, speak, or breathe"

Rescuer shouts "Help!"

☐ ☐ **Perform Abdominal Thrusts**

– Stand behind victim

– Wrap arms around victim's waist

– Make a fist with one hand and place thumb side of fist against middle of victim's abdomen just above navel and well below lower tip of breastbone

– Grasp your fist with your other hand

– Keeping elbows out, press fist into victim's abdomen with a quick upward thrust

– Each thrust should be a separate and distinct attempt to dislodge the object

– Repeat thrusts until obstruction is cleared or victim becomes unconscious

Final Instructor Check_____

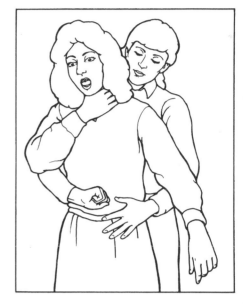

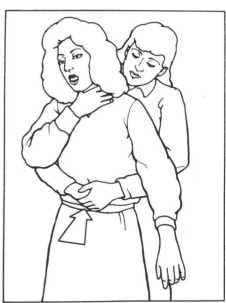

Skill Sheet

You find a person lying on the ground, not moving. You should survey the scene to see if it is safe and to get some idea of what happened. Then begin doing a primary survey by checking the ABCs.

Remember: **Do not perform finger sweeps on a manikin. Do not touch the manikin's lips or inside the mouth with your finger.**

Partner Check   Instructor Check

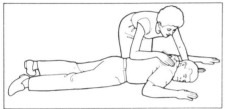

☐ ☐ **Check for Unresponsiveness**

Tap or gently shake victim

Rescuer shouts "Are you OK?"

Partner/Instructor says "Unconscious"

Rescuer repeats "Unconscious"

Rescuer shouts "Help!"

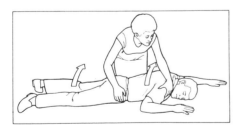

☐ ☐ **Position the Victim**

– Roll victim onto back, if necessary

Kneel facing victim, midway between victim's hips and shoulders

Straighten victim's legs, if necessary, and move arm closest to you above victim's head

Lean over victim, and place one hand on victim's shoulder and other hand on victim's hip

Roll victim toward you as a single unit; as you roll victim, move your hand from shoulder to support back of head and neck

Place victim's arm nearest you alongside victim's body

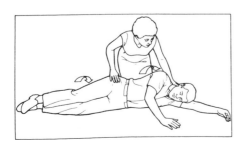

Partner Check

Instructor Check

☐ ☐ **Open the Airway:** Use head-tilt/chin-lift method

Place one hand on victim's forehead

– Place fingers of other hand under bony part of lower jaw near chin

– Tilt head and lift jaw—avoid closing victim's mouth

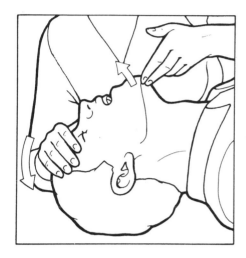

☐ ☐ **Check for Breathlessness**

– Maintain open airway

– Place your ear over victim's mouth and nose

– Look at chest, listen and feel for breathing for 3 to 5 seconds

Partner/Instructor says "No breathing"

Rescuer repeats "No breathing"

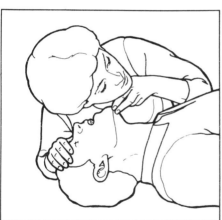

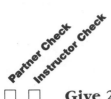

☐ ☐ **Give 2 Full Breaths**

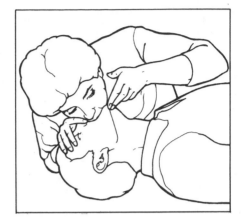

– Maintain open airway

– Pinch nose shut

– Open your mouth wide, take a deep breath, and make a tight seal around outside of victim's mouth

– Give 2 full breaths at the rate of 1 to 1½ seconds per breath

Partner/Instructor says "Unable to breathe air into victim"

☐ ☐ **Retilt Victim's Head and Give 2 Full Breaths**

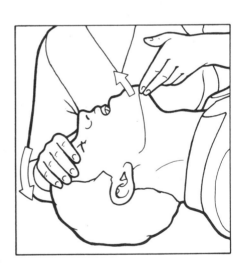

– Retilt victim's head

– Pinch nose shut

– Open your mouth wide, take a deep breath, and make a tight seal around outside of victim's mouth

– Give 2 full breaths at the rate of 1 to 1½ seconds per breath

Partner/Instructor says "Still unable to breathe air into victim"

Rescuer says "Airway obstructed"

☐ ☐ **Phone the EMS System for Help**

– Tell someone to call for an ambulance

Rescuer says "Airway obstructed, call _____"
(Local emergency number or Operator)

☐ ☐ **Perform 6 to 10 Abdominal Thrusts**

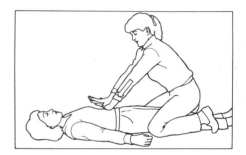

– Straddle victim's thighs

– Place heel of one hand against middle of victim's
abdomen just above navel and well below lower tip
of breastbone

– Place other hand directly on top of first hand
(fingers of both hands should be pointing toward
victim's head)

– Press into victim's abdomen 6 to 10 times with
quick upward thrusts

– Each thrust should be a separate and distinct
attempt to dislodge the object

Partner Check

Instructor Check

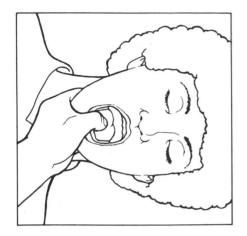

☐ ☐ **Do Finger Sweep (Pretend)**

- Move from straddle position and kneel beside victim's head

- With victim's face up, open the mouth and grasp both tongue and lower jaw between thumb and fingers of hand nearest victim's legs; lift jaw

- Insert index finger into mouth along inside of cheek and deep into throat to base of tongue

- Use "hooking" action to dislodge object and move it into mouth for removal

Partner/Instructor says "No object found"

Rescuer repeats "No object found"

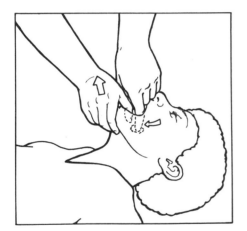

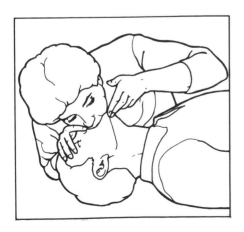

☐ ☐ **Give 2 Full Breaths**

- Open airway

- Pinch nose shut

- Open your mouth wide, take a deep breath, and make a tight seal around outside of victim's mouth

- Give 2 full breaths at the rate of 1 to 1½ seconds per breath

If airway is still blocked, say "Airway still obstructed"

Partner Check Instructor Check

☐ ☐ **Repeat Sequence**

– Do 6 to 10 abdominal thrusts

– Do finger sweep (pretend)

– Attempt to give breaths

☐ ☐ **What to Do Next**

While the rescuer is repeating the sequence of abdominal thrusts, finger sweep, and rescue breaths, the partner should read one of the following statements:

1. Rescuer can breathe into victim's lungs after doing finger sweep.

2. Object is removed during finger sweep.

3. Object is expelled during abdominal thrusts.

Based on this information, the rescuer should make a decision about what to do next, and continue to give the right care.

Final Instructor Check_____

First Aid for Choking When a Conscious Victim Becomes Unconscious

If a victim who is choking loses consciousness while you are giving abdominal or chest thrusts, you should shout for help and slowly lower the victim to the floor while supporting the victim from behind. Make sure the victim's head doesn't hit the floor.

Once you have lowered the victim to the floor, have someone phone the EMS system for help if it hasn't already been done.

1. Do a finger sweep.
2. Open the airway and give two full breaths.
3. Give 6 to 10 abdominal thrusts if you are unable to breathe air into the victim's lungs.

Repeat these three steps (finger sweep, rescue breaths, 6 to 10 abdominal thrusts) in the same sequence until the obstruction is cleared or until EMS personnel arrive and take over.

If You Are Alone and Choking

If you are choking and there is no one around to help, you can do an abdominal thrust on yourself. Make a fist with one hand and place the thumb side on the middle of your abdomen slightly above the navel and well below the tip of your breastbone. Grasp your fist with your other hand and give a quick upward thrust. You can also lean forward and press your abdomen over any firm, non-sharp object such as the back of a chair, a railing, or a sink.

What to Do for Heart Attack

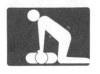

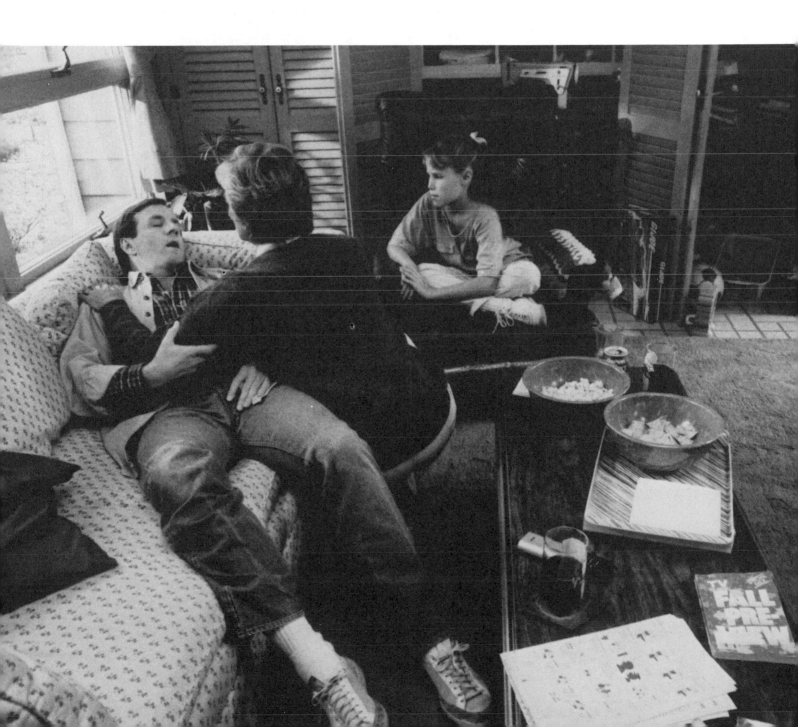

In this chapter you will learn what a heart attack is and what to do for someone who is having a heart attack. You will also learn what you can do to prevent heart attack. In order to give a heart attack victim the best chance of surviving, you must first be able to **recognize** the signals of a heart attack. This isn't always easy. Once you recognize the signals, you must then give the correct first aid.

Objectives

By the time you finish reading this chapter, you should be able to to the following:

1. List three signals of a heart attack.
2. Describe why it is important to know that heart attack victims often deny that they are having a heart attack.
3. Describe the first aid for a heart attack.
4. List the risk factors for cardiovascular disease.

What Is a Heart Attack?

A heart attack happens when one or more of the blood vessels that supply blood to a portion of the heart become blocked. When this happens, the blood can't get through to feed that part of the heart. When the flow of oxygen-carrying blood is cut off, the cells of this part of the heart begin to die. This is what happens during a heart attack. The heart may not be able to pump properly because part of it is dying.

If a large part of the heart is not getting blood, then the heart may not be able to pump at all. If the heart stops, it is called **cardiac arrest.**

Since any heart attack may lead to cardiac arrest, it is important to be able to recognize when someone is having a heart attack. Prompt action may prevent the victim's heart from stopping. The simple truth is that a heart attack victim whose heart is still beating has a far better chance of living than someone whose heart has stopped. Most people who die from a heart attack die within one to two hours after the first signals of the heart attack occur. Many of these people could be saved if bystanders were able to recognize the signals of a heart attack and take prompt action.

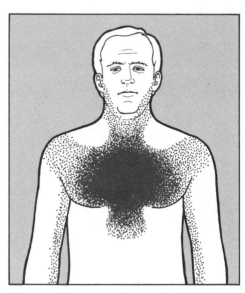

Figure 32
Areas for Heart Attack Pain

Signals of a Heart Attack

The most significant signal of a heart attack is chest discomfort or pain. A victim may describe it as uncomfortable pressure, squeezing, a fullness or tightness, aching, crushing, constricting, oppressive, or heavy. The pain is described as being in the center of the chest behind the breastbone. The pain may spread to one or both shoulders or arms, or to the neck, jaw, or back *(Fig. 32)*.

In addition to chest pain there may be other signals, including:

- Sweating
- Nausea
- Shortness of breath.

Many victims deny that they are having a heart attack. They may not want to admit to themselves or to others that they are having a heart attack. This may delay medical care when it is needed most. Heart attack victims may deny that they are having a heart attack by saying, for example, "I'm too healthy," or, "It's indigestion or something I ate," or, "It can't happen to me," or, "I don't want to bother my doctor," or, "This is something I can take care of myself," or, "I don't want to frighten anyone," or, "I'll feel ridiculous bothering everybody if it isn't a heart attack." These excuses are a signal to take immediate action.

First Aid for Heart Attacks

1. Recognize the signals of a heart attack and take action.
2. Have the victim stop what he or she is doing and sit or lie down in a comfortable position. Do not let the victim move around.
3. Have someone phone the emergency medical services (EMS) system for help. If you are alone, you phone.

A key factor in whether or not a victim will survive a heart attack is how quickly the victim receives advanced care. Therefore, it is important that you call the EMS system right away.

Not all ambulances are staffed and equipped to provide advanced care to the victim at the scene of an emergency, but in most cases it is better to call for an ambulance to transport the victim, rather than to transport the victim in a private vehicle yourself. The victim's condition could worsen on the way to the hospital, and an ambulance is equipped and staffed to deal with conditions that could develop during the transport. In addition, transporting a victim in a private vehicle places tremendous emotional pressures on the driver. This puts **all** occupants of the vehicle at added risk.

What to Do for Heart Attack

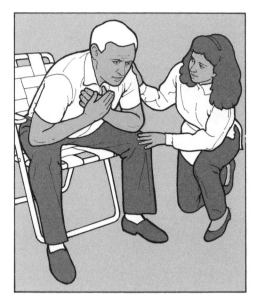

Figure 33
Caring for the Heart Attack Victim

There may be some situations, however, when an ambulance is not readily available, and you may have to weigh the risks and consider driving the victim to the hospital. You should know that not all hospitals and health facilities offer advanced care for cardiac emergencies, nor do they all offer it on a 24-hour basis. Therefore, it is important to be familiar with the emergency resources of your community, and know your plan of action **before** an emergency happens.

After the EMS system has been called, you should ask the victim for information about his or her condition *(Fig. 33).* Bystanders may also be of help here; they may be able to give you some of this information. The questions you should ask as part of this interview are explained in Chapter 2, "How to Deal With an Emergency." You should try to get the following information:

- Victim's name.
- Victim's age.
- Previous medical problems. ("Has anything like this ever happened to you before?")
- Where it hurts and how long the person has had pain.
- Type of pain (for example, "dull," "heavy," "sharp").

Because the heart attack victim's heart may stop beating, you should be prepared to give CPR.

Review Questions

Fill in the blanks with the right word(s), and check the best answer.

1. What is the most significant signal of a heart attack?

_____.

2. What is the first aid for a heart attack?

    a. Recognize the _____ of a heart attack.

    b. Make the victim _____ or

    _____ down in a comfortable position.

    c. Call the _____ system for help.

3. As you are walking home from work, you notice your neighbor sitting in her car in her driveway. She explains that she is having pain in her chest and asks you to help her into her house. Which of the following should you **not** do if possible?

    ☐ a. Help her walk to the house.
    ☐ b. Tell her to rest where she is.

Answers

1. Chest discomfort or pain is the most significant signal of a heart attack.

2. The first aid for a heart attack is to:

 a. Recognize the **signals** of a heart attack.
 b. Make the victim **sit or lie** down in a comfortable position.
 c. Call the **EMS** system for help.

3. a. You should **not help her walk to the house.** (A person who is having chest pain should not move around.)

How Heart Attacks Happen

While heart attacks seem to strike suddenly, the conditions that often cause them may build up silently for years. Most heart attacks are the result of **cardiovascular disease.** Cardiovascular disease happens when fatty substances and other materials build up in the blood and begin to stick to the walls of the blood vessels. Over time, the blood vessels get narrower. As the blood vessels get narrower, it becomes more and more likely that a blood vessel in the heart will become partly or completely clogged *(Fig. 34).* This process can begin in early life; some scientists believe it may even begin in early childhood.

Most of the people in this room may have some form of cardiovascular disease. Cardiovascular disease may only be stopped or slowed by certain changes in the way you live. This disease cannot be stopped by medicines, though some related problems (like high blood pressure) can be controlled or slowed by medicines.

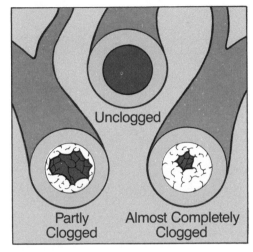

Figure 34
Clogged Arteries

Risk Factors

Scientists have been able to identify certain things that are related to getting cardiovascular disease. They call these **risk factors.** In this course, there is not enough time to give you a lot of information about risk factors, but we have included the list below so that you can see which apply to you.

Risk Factors That You Cannot Change

- Heredity (a history of cardiovascular disease in your family).
- Sex (males are at greater risk).
- Age (you are at greater risk as you get older).
- Race (blacks are at greater risk for cardiovascular disease).

Risk Factors That You Can Change

- Cigarette smoking.
- High blood pressure.
- High blood cholesterol (influenced by a diet high in saturated fat and cholesterol).
- Uncontrolled diabetes.
- Obesity (overweight).
- Lack of exercise.
- Stress.

Some of you will be motivated by this list to take action, while others will not. Unfortunately, there is no quick fix for dealing with the risk of cardiovascular disease. **Just reading the list won't reduce your risk of having a heart attack.** Reducing your risk requires effort on your part and guidance from your doctor or health care provider.

If you are interested in learning more about how to reduce your risk of cardiovascular disease, the American Red Cross can tell you about the resources available in your community to help you.

Review Questions

Fill in the blanks with the right word(s).

4. When a person has cardiovascular disease, over time that person's blood vessels get _____.

5. Blood vessels become clogged when _____ substances and other materials begin to stick to the walls of the blood vessels.

6. Most heart attacks happen when blood vessels become clogged and cut off the flow of _____ to the heart.

7. What are the risk factors for cardiovascular disease that you cannot change?

   1. Heredity (a history of cardiovascular disease in your _____).
   2. Sex (_____ are at greater risk).
   3. Age (you are at greater risk as you get _____).
   4. Race (_____ are at greater risk).

8. What are seven risk factors that you can work on to reduce your risk of cardiovascular disease?

   1. Cigarette smoking.
   2. _____ blood pressure.
   3. High blood cholesterol.
   4. Lack of _____.
   5. Obesity or being _____.
   6. Uncontrolled diabetes.
   7. Stress.

Answers

4. When a person has cardiovascular disease, over time that person's blood vessels get **narrower.**

5. Blood vessels become clogged when **fatty** substances and other materials begin to stick to the walls of the blood vessels.

6. Most heart attacks happen when blood vessels become clogged and cut off the flow of **blood** to the heart.

7. The risk factors for cardiovascular disease that you cannot change are:

    1. Heredity (a history of cardiovascular disease in your **family**).
    2. Sex (**males** are at greater risk).
    3. Age (you are at greater risk as you get **older**).
    4. Race (**blacks** are at greater risk).

8. The seven risk factors that you can work on to reduce your risk of cardiovascular disease are:

    1. Cigarette smoking.
    2. **High** blood pressure.
    3. High blood cholesterol.
    4. Lack of **exercise**.
    5. Obesity or being **overweight**.
    6. Uncontrolled diabetes.
    7. Stress.

6

What to Do When the Heart Stops (CPR)

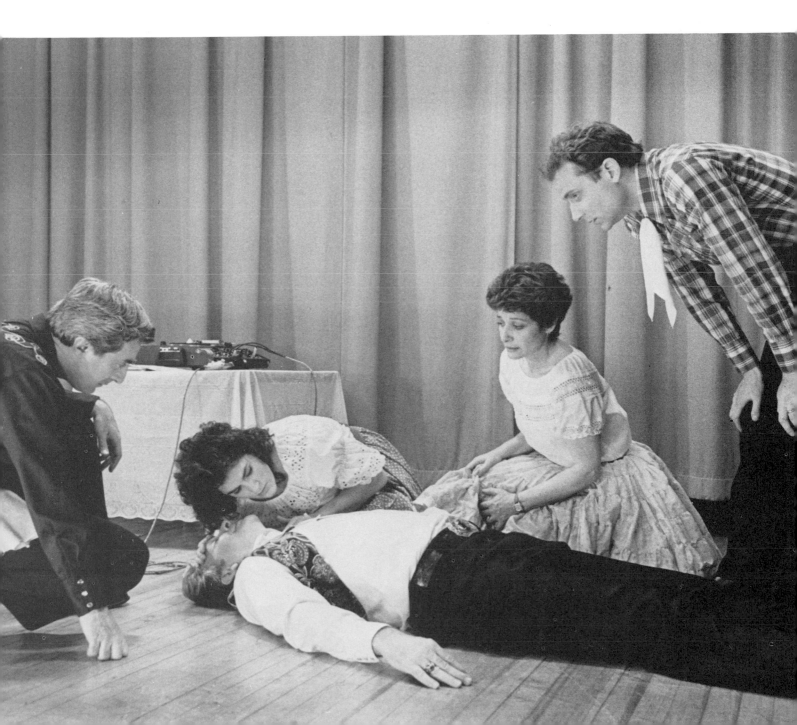

In this chapter you will find out what to do for someone whose heart has stopped beating. You will learn how to keep oxygen-carrying blood moving through the victim's body.

Cardiopulmonary resuscitation (CPR) is a combination of chest compressions and rescue breathing. "Cardio" refers to the heart and "pulmonary" refers to the lungs. When you give CPR, you do chest compressions and rescue breathing together. This supplies oxygen to the victim's blood and moves the blood through the body to supply the cells with oxygen.

A Look at the Heart

The heart is a tough muscular organ about the size of your fist. It is located roughly in the center of the chest between your lungs and under the lower half of the breastbone. The heart is protected in the front by the ribs and breastbone and in the back by the backbone.

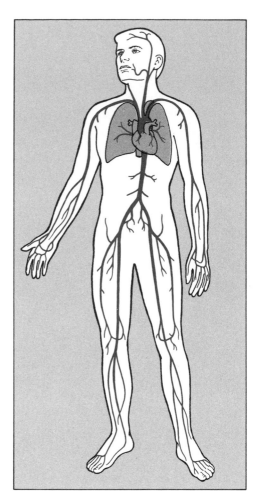

Figure 35
The Heart and Major Blood Vessels

The heart pumps blood to all parts of your body through blood vessels. Blood vessels are the tubes that carry blood to the cells of the body. How well this system works depends on the condition of your blood vessels and your heart *(Fig. 35)*.

For the average adult, the heart pumps about 70 times each minute, or about 100,000 times each day. In the minute or so it takes you to read this section, your heart has pumped more than a gallon of blood. If a person's heart should stop beating, that person needs help immediately to keep oxygen-carrying blood flowing to the body's cells until EMS personnel arrive.

Review Questions

Fill in the blanks with the right word(s).

1. The purpose of the heart is to _____
   blood to all parts of the body.

2. How well your circulatory system works depends on the
   condition of your _____ and your blood
   _____.

Answers

1. The purpose of the heart is to **pump** blood to all parts of the body.

2. How well your circulatory system works depends on the condition of your **heart** and your blood **vessels**.

The Purpose of CPR and Why It Works

To help a person in cardiac arrest, you must provide CPR. CPR has two purposes. By breathing into the victim and compressing the chest, you:

1. Keep the lungs supplied with oxygen when breathing has stopped.
2. Keep blood circulating and carrying oxygen to the brain, heart, and other parts of the body.

All of your body's living cells need a steady supply of oxygen to keep you alive. CPR must be started as soon as possible after the heart stops. Any delay in starting CPR reduces the chances that EMS personnel will be able to restart the heart. In addition, brain cells begin to die after four to six minutes without oxygen.

Review Questions

Fill in the blanks with the right word(s).

3. The two purposes of CPR are:

   a. To keep the lungs supplied with _____ when the respiratory system has failed.

   b. To keep _____ circulating and carrying _____ to the brain, heart, and other parts of the body.

4. CPR must be started as soon as possible to increase the chances that EMS personnel will be able to _____ the heart.

Answers

3. The two purposes of CPR are:
   a. To keep the lungs supplied with **oxygen** when the respiratory system has failed.
   b. To keep the **blood** circulating and carrying **oxygen** to the brain, heart, and other parts of the body.

4. CPR must be started as soon as possible to increase the chances that EMS personnel will be able to **restart** the heart.

How to Give CPR

In order to find out if a person needs CPR, you begin with a primary survey to check the ABCs as you did for rescue breathing. You should:

1. Check for unresponsiveness.
2. Shout for help.
3. Position the victim on his or her back.
4. Open the airway.
5. Look, listen, and feel for breathing.
6. If the victim is not breathing, give two full breaths.
7. Check the carotid pulse.
8. Have someone phone the EMS system for help.

If there is no pulse, you will have to give CPR. **It is important that you check the victim's carotid pulse for 5 to 10 seconds before starting CPR because it is dangerous to perform chest compressions if the heart is beating.**

To give CPR, the rescuer kneels beside the victim, leans over the chest, and presses down and comes up at a steady pace. Chest compressions are alternated with rescue breaths. These actions keep oxygen-carrying blood flowing through the blood vessels.

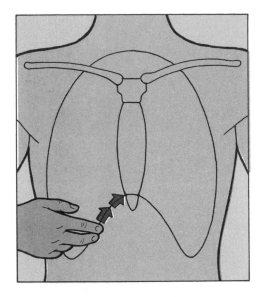

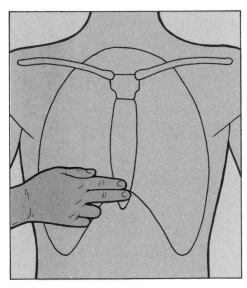

Figure 36
Find Correct Position

Locating the Compression Position

For chest compressions to work, the victim must be lying flat on his or her back on a firm, flat surface. The victim's head must be on the same level as the heart. In order to give effective compressions, your hands and body must be in the right place.

- Kneel facing the victim's chest with your knees against the victim.
- Using the hand nearest the victim's legs, find the lower edge of the rib cage on the side closest to you. Run your middle and index fingers up the edge of the rib cage to the "notch" where the ribs meet the breastbone in the center of the lower part of the chest *(Fig. 36)*. With your middle finger on this "notch," place the index finger of the same hand next to it on the lower end of the breastbone.

- Place the heel of your other hand on the breastbone right next to the index finger of the hand you used to find the "notch." The heel of your hand should rest along the length of the breastbone *(Fig. 37)*.
- Once the heel of your hand is in position on the chest, remove the other hand from the "notch" and place the heel of this hand directly on top of the heel of the hand already on the victim's breastbone *(Fig. 38)*.

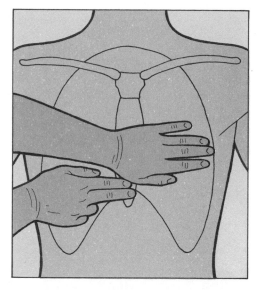

Figure 37
Place Heel of Hand on Breastbone

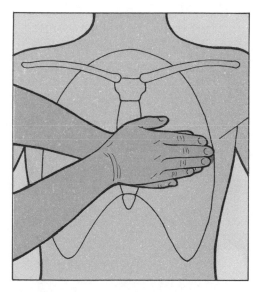

Figure 38
Place Second Hand over Heel of First

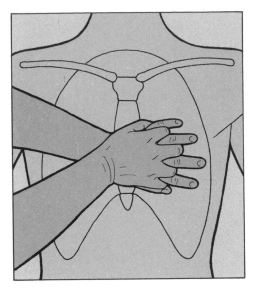

Figure 39
Interlace Fingers

- Keep your fingers off the victim's chest. To do this you may interlace them or hold them upward *(Fig. 39)*.
- Finding the correct hand position in this way allows you to compress right on the breastbone, and keeps hand pressure off the ribs and away from the tip of the breastbone. This will decrease the chance of fracturing the ribs which are on either side of the breastbone. It will also keep you from pushing the tip of the breastbone into the delicate organs beneath it.
- Another acceptable hand position, for people with arthritic conditions, is to grasp the wrist of the hand on the chest with the hand that located the "notch" at the lower end of the breastbone *(Fig. 40)*.

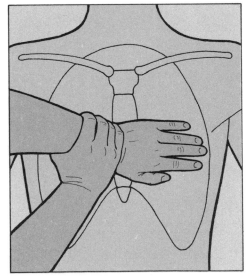

Figure 40
Alternate Hand Placement

Review Questions

Check the best answers.

5. Which of the following surfaces would be good for giving CPR? (Check all that apply.)
   - ☐ a. Bed
   - ☐ b. Floor
   - ☐ c. Ground.

6. The first step in finding the proper hand position to give chest compressions is to:
   - ☐ a. Run your middle and index fingers up the edge of the rib cage to the "notch" where the ribs meet the breastbone.
   - ☐ b. Find the top of the breastbone.
   - ☐ c. Find the navel.

7. When your hands are in the correct position to give CPR, where should your fingers be?
   - ☐ a. Resting on the victim's chest.
   - ☐ b. Held off the victim's chest.
   - ☐ c. Curling into your palm.

Answers

5. When you give CPR, the victim should be on a hard surface such as:
b. the **floor**, or
c. the **ground**.

6. a. The first step in finding the proper hand position to give chest compressions is to **run your middle and index fingers up the edge of the rib cage to the "notch" where the ribs meet the breastbone.**

7. b. When your hands are in the correct position to give CPR, your fingers should be **held off the victim's chest.**

Body Position of Rescuer

The position of the rescuer's body is very important when giving compressions. While keeping your hands in the correct position and kneeling facing the victim's chest, straighten your arms and lock your elbows so that your shoulders are directly over your hands. In this position, when you push down, you will be pushing straight down onto the breastbone. The weight of your upper body creates the pressure necessary to compress the chest *(Fig. 41)*.

Compression Technique

Here is the technique for giving chest compressions:

1. When you compress, you push with the weight of your body, not with the muscles of your arms. Push straight down. If you rock back and forth and don't push straight down, your compressions will not be effective *(Fig. 42)*.

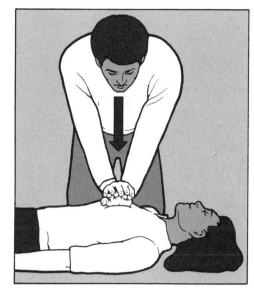

Figure 41
Correct Position of Rescuer

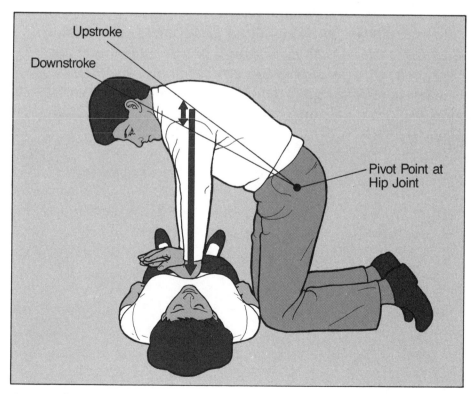

Upstroke

Downstroke

Pivot Point at Hip Joint

Figure 42
Correct Position of Rescuer

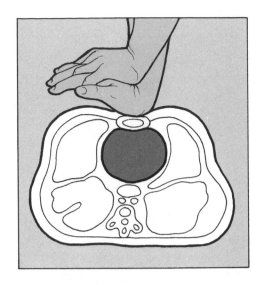

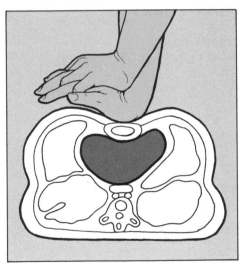

Figure 43
Compress Chest 1½ to 2 Inches

2. Each compression should push the breastbone down from 1½ to 2 inches (3.8 to 5 centimeters) *(Fig. 43)*.

The downward and upward movement should be smooth, not jerky. Maintain a steady down and up rhythm and do not pause between compressions. Half the time should be spent pushing down and half the time should be spent coming up. Release pressure on the chest completely but don't let your hands lose contact with the chest, or lose their correct position on the breastbone.

3. Give compressions at the rate of 80 to 100 compressions per minute.
4. If your hands lose contact with the chest, you should reposition them before compressing again. Find the "notch" as you did before, in order to position your hands correctly.

Compression/Breathing Cycles

When you give CPR, you will do cycles of 15 compressions and 2 breaths. In each cycle, you will give 15 compressions and then open the airway and give 2 full breaths.

Each time you begin a new cycle of compressions and breaths, locate the correct hand position for compressions using the "notch."

Review Questions

Check the best answer.

8. When you give CPR, your arms should be:
   - ☐ a. Bent.
   - ☐ b. Straight.

9. How far do you compress the chest of an adult?
   - ☐ a. 1 inch to 1½ inches (2.5 to 3.8 centimeters).
   - ☐ b. 1½ to 2 inches (3.8 to 5 centimeters).
   - ☐ c. 2 to 3 inches (5 to 7.6 centimeters).

10. At what rate should you compress the chest during CPR?
    - ☐ a. 50 to 60 times per minute.
    - ☐ b. 60 to 80 times per minute.
    - ☐ c. 80 to 100 times per minute.

11. What should you do if your hands move out of position while compressing the chest?
    - ☐ a. Continue compressions.
    - ☐ b. Reposition your hands by locating the "notch" and continue compressions.
    - ☐ c. Place your hands back where they were but do not waste time by relocating the "notch."

Answers

8. b. When you give CPR, your arms should be **straight.**

9. b. You compress the chest of an adult 1½ **to 2 inches** (3.8 to 5 centimeters).

10. c. During CPR, compress the chest at the rate of **80 to 100 times per minute.**

11. b. If your hands move out of position, **reposition your hands by relocating the "notch" and continue compressions.**

Putting the Steps Together

Here are the steps you should follow when you give CPR:

1. Check for unresponsiveness. Tap or gently shake the victim and shout, "Are you OK?"

2. Shout for help.

3. Position the victim.

4. Open the airway.

5. Look, listen, and feel for breathing (3 to 5 seconds).

6. If the victim is not breathing, give two full breaths.

7. Check the victim's carotid pulse for heartbeat (5 to 10 seconds).

8. Tell someone to phone the EMS system for help.

9. If there is no pulse, find the correct hand position and position your body to give compressions.

10. Give 15 compressions without stopping, at the rate of 80 to 100 per minute, counting out loud, "One and two and three and four and five and six and seven and eight and nine and ten and eleven and twelve and thirteen and fourteen and fifteen and." Push down as you say the number and come up as you say the "and."

11. Next, quickly tilt the victim's head back and lift the jaw, and give 2 full breaths to the victim the same way you gave the first 2 breaths.

12. Keep repeating—15 compressions, 2 breaths, 15 compressions, 2 breaths, and so on. The complete cycle of 15 compressions and 2 breaths should take from 11 to 14 seconds *(Fig. 44)*.

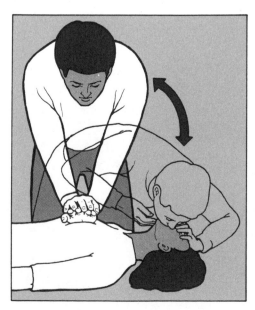

Figure 44
15 Compressions, then 2 Breaths

13. Recheck pulse. After doing four cycles (or about one minute) of continuous CPR, you should check to see if the victim has a pulse.

    Do this after giving the 2 breaths at the end of the fourth cycle of 15 compressions and 2 breaths. Tilt the victim's head back and check the carotid pulse for 5 seconds.

    If there is no pulse, give 2 breaths and continue CPR (compressions and rescue breaths). Repeat these pulse checks every few minutes.

    If you do find a pulse, then check for breathing for 3 to 5 seconds. If breathing is present, keep the airway open and monitor breathing and pulse closely. This means that you should look, listen, and feel for breathing while you keep checking the pulse. If there is no breathing, perform rescue breathing and keep checking the pulse.

14. Continue to give CPR until one of the following things happens:

    - The heart starts beating again and the victim begins breathing.
    - A second rescuer trained in CPR takes over for you.
    - EMS personnel arrive and take over.
    - You are too exhausted to continue.

Review Questions

Check the best answer, and fill in the blanks with the right word(s).

12. When you perform CPR, what is the ratio of compressions to breaths?
☐ a. 10 compressions, then 1 breath.
☐ b. 15 compressions, then 2 breaths.
☐ c. 12 compressions, then 15 breaths.

13. After starting CPR, how often should you check for the return of pulse?
☐ a. After 5 minutes and every 5 to 6 minutes thereafter.
☐ b. After 2 minutes and every 4 to 5 minutes thereafter.
☐ c. After 1 minute and every few minutes thereafter.

14. What are the four conditions when you may stop CPR?

a. When the heart starts _____ again.

b. When a second rescuer trained in

_____ takes over for you.

c. When _____ personnel arrive and take

over.

d. When you are too _____ to continue.

Answers

12. b. When you perform CPR, the ratio is **15 compressions, then 2 breaths.**

13. c. After starting CPR, check for the return of pulse **after 1 minute and every few minutes thereafter.**

14. You may stop CPR:
  a. When the heart starts **beating** again.
  b. When a second rescuer trained in **CPR** takes over for you.
  c. When **EMS** personnel arrive and take over.
  d. When you are too **exhausted** to continue.

Practice Session: Adult CPR

The CPR practice session is the last of the three practice sessions. During this session, you and a partner will practice only on a manikin.

Before you start practicing, carefully read the skill sheet checklist on pages 130 through 138 in this workbook.

Skill Sheet

You find a person lying on the ground, not moving. You should survey the scene to see if it is safe and to get some idea of what happened. Then begin doing a primary survey by checking the ABCs.

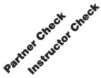

Partner Check   Instructor Check

☐ ☐ **Check for Unresponsiveness**

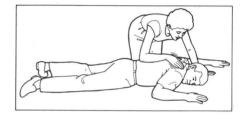

Tap or gently shake victim

Rescuer shouts "Are you OK?"

Partner/Instructor says "Unconscious"

Rescuer says "Unconscious"

Rescuer shouts "Help!"

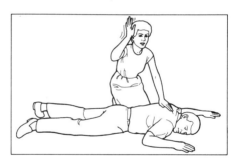

☐ ☐ **Position the Victim**

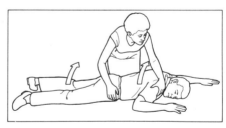

– Roll victim onto back, if necessary

Kneel facing victim, midway between victim's hips and shoulders

Lean over victim, and place one hand on victim's shoulder and other hand on victim's hip

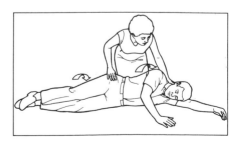

Roll victim toward you as a single unit; as you roll victim, move your hand from shoulder to support back of head and neck

Place victim's arm nearest you alongside victim's body

Partner Check   Instructor Check

☐ ☐ **Open the Airway:** Use head-tilt/chin-lift method

Place one hand on victim's forehead

– Place fingers of other hand under bony part of lower jaw near chin

– Tilt head and lift jaw—avoid closing victim's mouth

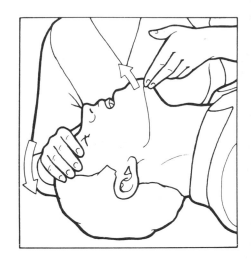

☐ ☐ **Check for Breathlessness**

– Maintain open airway

– Place your ear over victim's mouth and nose

– Look at chest, listen and feel for breathing for 3 to 5 seconds

Partner/Instructor says "No breathing"

Rescuer repeats "No breathing"

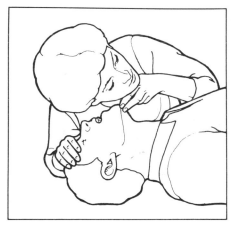

☐ ☐ **Give 2 Full Breaths**

– Maintain open airway

– Pinch nose shut

– Open your mouth wide, take a deep breath, and make a tight seal around outside of victim's mouth

– Give 2 full breaths at the rate of 1 to 1½ seconds per breath

– Observe chest rise and fall; listen and feel for escaping air

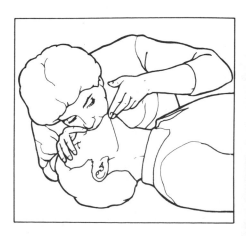

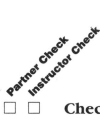

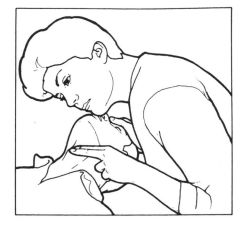

☐ ☐ **Check for Pulse**

- Maintain head tilt with one hand on forehead

- Locate Adam's apple with middle and index fingers of hand closest to victim's feet

- Slide fingers down into groove of neck on side closest to you

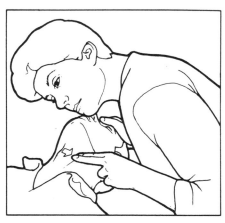

- Feel for carotid pulse for 5 to 10 seconds

Partner/Instructor says "No breathing and no pulse"

Rescuer repeats "No breathing and no pulse"

☐ ☐ **Phone the EMS System for Help**

- Tell someone to call for an ambulance

Rescuer says "No breathing, no pulse, call _____." (Local emergency number or Operator)

☐ ☐ **Locate Compression Position**

– Kneel facing victim's chest

– With middle and index fingers of hand nearest victim's legs, locate lower edge of victim's rib cage on side closest to you

– Follow rib cage to "notch" at lower end of breastbone

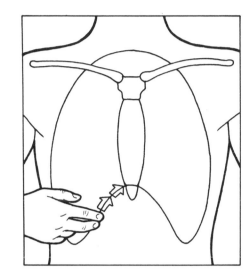

– Place middle finger in "notch," and index finger next to it on the lower end of breastbone

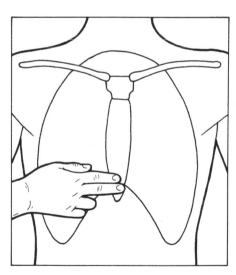

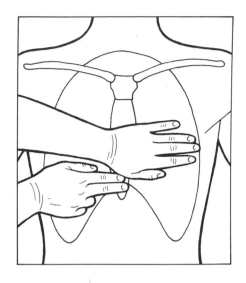

– Place heel of hand nearest victim's head on breastbone next to index finger of hand used to find "notch"

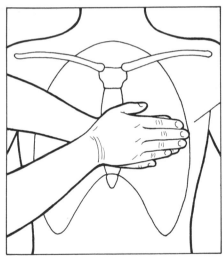

– Place heel of hand used to locate "notch" directly on top of heel of other hand

– Keep fingers off victim's chest

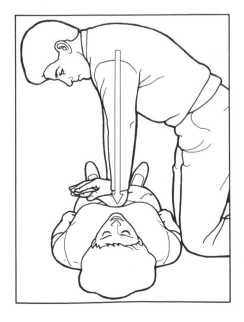

– Position shoulders over hands with elbows locked and arms straight

☐ ☐ **Give 15 Compressions**

– Compress breastbone 1½ to 2 inches (3.8 to 5 centimeters) at a rate of 80 to 100 compressions per minute (15 compressions should take 9 to 11 seconds)

Count aloud "One and two and three and four and five and six and . . . . fifteen and" (Push down as you say the number and come up as you say "and")

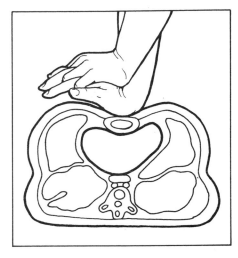

– Compress down and up smoothly, keeping hand contact with chest at all times

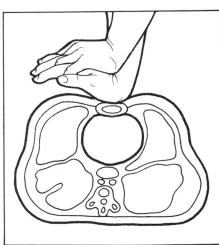

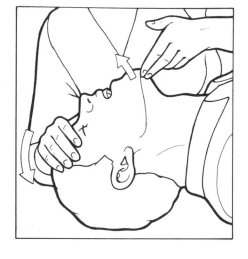

Partner Check   Instructor Check

☐ ☐ **Give 2 Full Breaths**

- Open airway

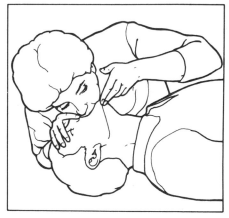

- Pinch nose shut

- Open your mouth wide, take a deep breath, and make a tight seal around outside of victim's mouth

- Give 2 full breaths at the rate of 1 to 1½ seconds per breath

- Observe chest rise and fall; listen and feel for escaping air

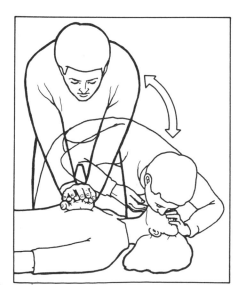

☐ ☐ **Do Compression/Breathing Cycles**

- Do 4 cycles of 15 compressions and 2 breaths

Partner Check
Instructor Check

☐ ☐ **Recheck Pulse**

– Tilt head

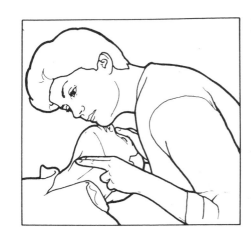

– Locate carotid pulse and feel for 5 seconds

Partner/Instructor says "No pulse"

Rescuer repeats "No pulse"

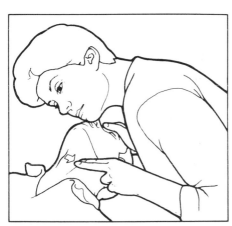

☐ ☐ **Give 2 Full Breaths**

– Open airway

– Pinch nose shut

– Open your mouth wide and make a tight seal around outside of victim's mouth

– Give 2 full breaths at the rate of 1 to 1½ seconds per breath

– Observe chest rise and fall; listen and feel for escaping air

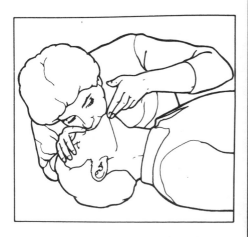

Partner Check
Instructor Check

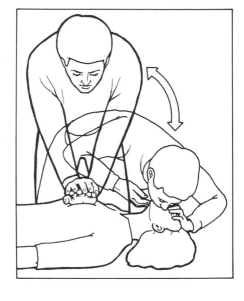

☐ ☐ **Continue Compression/Breathing Cycles**

– Locate correct hand position

– Continue cycles of 15 compressions and 2 breaths

Recheck pulse every few minutes

☐ ☐ **What to Do Next**

When the rescuer stops to check pulse, the partner should read one of the following statements:

1. Victim has a pulse.

2. Victim does not have a pulse.

Based on this information, the rescuer should make a decision about what to do next, and continue giving the right care.

Final Instructor Check_____

More About CPR

If a Second Trained Rescuer Is at the Scene

If another rescuer trained in CPR is at the scene, this person should do two things: first, phone the EMS system for help if this has not been done; second, take over CPR when the first rescuer is tired. Here are the steps for entry of the second rescuer:

- The second person should first identify himself or herself as a CPR-trained rescuer who is willing to help.
- If the EMS system has been called and if the first rescuer is tired and asks for help, then:

  1. The first rescuer should stop CPR after the next set of two breaths.
  2. The second rescuer should kneel next to the victim opposite the first rescuer, tilt the head back, and feel for the carotid pulse for five seconds.
  3. If there is no pulse, the second rescuer should give two breaths and continue CPR.
  4. The first rescuer should then check the adequacy of the second rescuer's breaths and chest compressions. This is done by watching the victim's chest rise and fall during rescue breathing, and by feeling the carotid pulse for an artificial pulse during chest compressions. This artificial pulse will tell you that blood is moving through the body.

If No One Comes When You Shout for Help

One of the first things you do when you discover an unresponsive victim is to shout for help. This is done to attract the attention of someone nearby who can phone the EMS system for help. But what if no one responds to your shouts for help? You should do CPR for at least one minute. During this minute you should continue to shout for help. You should also use this minute to plan how to make the call yourself.

If no one has responded to your shouts for help by the end of one minute of CPR, you should get to a phone as quickly as you can and phone the EMS system. Then quickly return to the victim and begin CPR again.

Notes

Review Section

Review Section

This section will help you review what you have learned in this course. You will be presented with a number of situations that you may find in real life. Fill in the blanks to tell what you would do if you came across these situations. The clues will help you make the correct decisions about what you should do.

Review Question: Rescue Breathing

You are walking past your neighbor's house and you hear shouts for help coming from the backyard. You run to the back of the house, and as you begin to survey the scene, you find your neighbor on the pool deck leaning over his wife. She is stretched out on her back and is not moving. Your neighbor says that one minute she was swimming, and the next minute she was floating face down in the water. What would you do next?

Do a primary survey to check the ABCs.

1. Check for _____. (See clue below)

2. Shout for _____.

3. Open the _____.

4. Look, listen, and feel for

   _____. (See clue)

5. Give two full _____.

6. Check for a _____. Where?

   _____. (See clue)

7. Have someone phone the _____

   _____ for help.

8. Begin _____ _____.

9. Give one breath every _____

   seconds. (See clue)

10. Keep the victim from moving until _____

    personnel arrive, and keep checking the victim's

    _____ and _____.

   CLUES: At step 1, the victim is unconscious.
   At step 4, the victim is not breathing.
   At step 6, the victim has a pulse.
   At step 9, after you have given rescue breaths for two
   minutes, the victim begins to breathe on her own.

Answers

1. Check for **unresponsiveness.**

2. Shout for **help.**

3. Open the **airway.**

4. Look, listen, and feel for **breathing.**

5. Give two full **breaths.**

6. Check for a **pulse at the side of the neck.**

7. Have someone phone the **EMS system** for help.

8. Begin **rescue breathing.**

9. Give one breath every **five** seconds.

10. Keep the victim from moving until **EMS** personnel arrive, and keep checking the victim's **breathing** and **pulse.**

Review Question: Recognizing the Signals of a Heart Attack

You are at a movie theater with your cousin and his wife. On the way out of the theater, your cousin stops and clutches his chest as if he is in great pain. When you ask him about it, he says he's fine, it's "just a little heartburn or indigestion." He is sweating and just doesn't look right. What would you do next?

1. Recognize the signals of a _____

   _____.

2. Make your cousin _____ or

   _____ down in a comfortable position.

3. Have someone phone the _____ system for help.

   NO CLUE NEEDED

Answers

1. Recognize the signals of a **heart attack.**

2. Make your cousin **sit** or **lie** down in a comfortable position.

3. Have someone phone the **EMS** system for help.

Review Question: CPR

You come to work early and find your boss lying face down on the floor in the office. She is not moving and there is no one else around. You survey the scene and see that it is safe to help her. What would you do next?

Do a primary survey to check the ABCs.

1. Check for _____. (See clue below)

2. Shout for _____.

3. Position the _____.

4. Open the _____.

5. Look, listen, and feel for _____. (See clue)

6. Give two full _____.

7. Check the carotid _____. (See clue)

8. Have someone phone the _____
   _____ for help.

9. Give CPR: cycles of _____ chest
   compressions and _____ rescue breaths.

10. After four cycles of CPR, check the carotid
    _____. (See clue)

11. Give _____ breaths.

12. Continue CPR until _____ personnel
    arrive and take over.

   CLUES: At step 1, the victim is unconscious.
   At step 5, the victim is not breathing.
   At step 7, the victim has no pulse.
   At step 10, the victim still has no pulse.

Answers

1. Check for **unresponsiveness.**

2. Shout for **help.**

3. Position the **victim.**

4. Open the **airway.**

5. Look, listen, and feel for **breathing.**

6. Give two full **breaths.**

7. Check the carotid **pulse.**

8. Have someone phone the **EMS system** for help.

9. Give CPR: cycles of **15** chest compressions and **2** rescue breaths.

10. After four cycles of CPR, check the carotid **pulse.**

11. Give **two** breaths.

12. Continue CPR until **EMS** personnel arrive and take over.

Review Question: Obstructed Airway

You go into a restroom at a shopping mall and find someone lying on the floor. You survey the scene and see that it is safe to help. What would you do next?

Do a primary survey to check the ABCs.

1. Check for _____. (See clue below)

2. Shout for _____.

3. Position the _____.

4. Open the _____.

5. Look, listen, and feel for _____. (See clue)

6. Give _____ _____
   _____. (See clue)

7. _____ the head.

8. Give _____ _____
   _____ again. (See clue)

9. Have someone phone the _____
   _____ for help.

10. Perform _____ to _____
    abdominal thrusts. (See clue)

11. Perform a _____ _____.
    (See clue)

12. Open the airway and give two _____
    _____. (See clue)

13. Keep the victim from moving until _____
    personnel arrive, and keep checking the victim's
    _____ and _____.

CLUES: At step 1, the victim is unconscious.
At step 5, the victim is not breathing.
At step 6, you are unable to breathe air into the victim.
At step 8, you are still unable to breathe air into the victim.
At step 10, you hear a gasp coming from the victim's
     mouth during the sixth thrust. You immediately stop
     giving thrusts.
At step 11, you find and remove a piece of food.
At step 12, victim begins breathing on his own.

Answers

1. Check for **unresponsiveness.**

2. Shout for **help.**

3. Position the **victim.**

4. Open the **airway.**

5. Look, listen, and feel for **breathing.**

6. Give **two full breaths.**

7. **Retilt** the head.

8. Give **two full breaths** again.

9. Have someone phone the **EMS system** for help.

10. Perform **6** to **10** abdominal thrusts.

11. Perform a **finger sweep.**

12. Open the airway and give two **full breaths.**

13. Keep the victim from moving until **EMS** personnel arrive, and keep checking the victim's **breathing** and **pulse.**

Appendix

Appendix — Information About Stroke

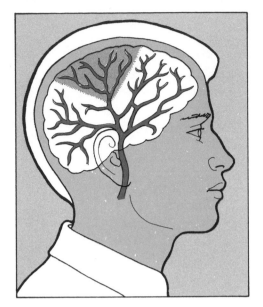

Figure 45
Stroke

The disease that causes most heart attacks can also cause stroke. When one of the vessels carrying blood to or through the brain bursts or becomes blocked by a clot, this may result in death to a part of the brain. If blood cannot get through to part of the brain, that part of the brain will not get enough oxygen and the brain cells will begin to die *(Fig. 45)*. This is called a **stroke.** It is similar to a heart attack, only it happens in the brain. As with a heart attack, your role is to recognize the signals and to take immediate action.

Objectives

By the time you finish reading this appendix, you should be able to do the following:

1. Describe the process that causes stroke.
2. List three signals of stroke.
3. Describe the first aid for stroke.

Signals of Stroke

Like the signals of a heart attack, the signals of a stroke may not be easy to recognize. Signals of a stroke may last from seconds to a few minutes to a few hours. The signals that you see will depend on the location of the damaged blood vessel and the amount of damage to the brain. The victim may show one or more of the following signals:

- Sudden, temporary weakness or numbness of the face, arm, or leg on one side of the body.
- Temporary loss of speech, or trouble speaking or understanding speech.
- Temporarily dimmed vision, or loss of vision, particularly in one eye.
- Unexplained dizziness, unsteadiness, or sudden falls.
- Severe headache.

First Aid for Stroke

Here are the steps you should follow:

1. Recognize the signals of a stroke and take action.

2. Have the victim stop what he or she is doing and rest in a comfortable position.

3. Do not let the victim eat or take medication.

4. Call the EMS system for help.

A key factor in whether or not a victim will survive a stroke is how quickly the victim receives advanced care. Therefore, it is important that you call the EMS system right away.

Not all ambulances are staffed and equipped to provide advanced care to the victim at the scene of an emergency, but in most cases it is better to call for an ambulance to transport the victim, rather than to transport the victim in a private vehicle yourself. The victim's condition could worsen on the way to the hospital, and an ambulance is equipped and staffed to deal with conditions that could develop during the transport. In addition, transporting a victim in a private vehicle places tremendous emotional pressures on the driver. This puts **all** occupants of the vehicle at added risk.

There may be some situations, however, when an ambulance is not readily available, and you may have to weigh the risks and consider driving the victim to the hospital. You should know that not all hospitals and health facilities offer advanced care, nor do they all offer it on a 24-hour basis. Therefore, it is important to be familiar with the emergency resources of your community, and know your plan of action **before** an emergency happens.

After the EMS system has been called, you should ask the victim and bystanders for information about the stroke victim's condition, as explained in Chapter 2, "How to Deal With an Emergency." You should try to get the following information:

- Victim's name
- Victim's age
- Previous medical problems ("Has anything like this ever happened to you before?")

If the victim becomes unconscious, position the victim on his or her back and monitor airway, breathing, and circulation. Should the victim vomit, turn the victim's head and body to the side and quickly wipe the material out of the victim's mouth. Keeping the victim positioned on his or her side, tilt the head back and monitor airway, breathing, and circulation.

Because the stroke victim's breathing and heart may stop, you should be prepared to give rescue breathing and CPR.

Review Questions

Check the best answer and fill in the blanks with the right word(s).

1. What happens when a person has a stroke?
    ☐ a. The flow of blood to part of the heart is blocked.
    ☐ b. The flow of blood to part of the brain is blocked.
    ☐ c. The flow of blood to the hands and feet is blocked.

2. Check three signals of stroke.

    ☐ a. Temporary loss of speech.
    ☐ b. Weakness or numbness on one side of the body.
    ☐ c. Crushing chest pain.
    ☐ d. Severe headache.

3. What is the first aid for stroke?

    1. _____ the signals and take action.

    2. Have the victim _____ in a comfortable position.

    3. Do not let the victim _____ or take

        _____.

    4. Phone the _____ system for help.

Answers

1. b. When a person has a stroke, **the flow of blood to part of the brain is blocked.**

2. Three signals of a stroke are:

   a. **Temporary loss of speech.**
   b. **Weakness or numbness on one side of the body.**
   d. **Severe headache.**

3. The first aid for stroke is:

   1. **Recognize** the signals and take action.
   2. Have the victim **rest** in a comfortable position.
   3. Do not let the victim **eat** or take **medication**.
   4. Phone the **EMS** system for help.

Appendix — The Emergency Medical Services (EMS) System

Throughout this course, you have learned how important it is for you and your community's EMS system to work together in order to give the victim of a medical emergency the best chance of survival.

This appendix explains what an EMS system is and how a victim of injury or sudden illness "enters" the system. It also explains the different types of care that a victim may require (basic life support and advanced life support) and what should happen when EMS personnel arrive at the scene of the emergency. At the end of this appendix there is a list of questions to help you learn more about your community's EMS system.

Objectives

By the time you finish reading this appendix, you should be able to:

1. Describe the purpose of an emergency medical services (EMS) system.

2. List at least three parts of an EMS system.

3. Describe the three main responsibilities of a trained citizen rescuer when a medical emergency occurs.

4. List five facts that you should know about your community's EMS system.

Appendix — The Emergency Medical Services (EMS) System

What Is an Emergency Medical Services (EMS) System?

To save a life in a life-threatening situation, two things must happen. Emergency care must be started right away by a trained bystander, and this care must be continued and enhanced by EMS personnel when they arrive. If no one with first aid training is nearby to begin emergency care immediately, or if the community's EMS system cannot quickly provide the right kind of help, then a victim's chances of survival may be greatly reduced.

By taking this course, you have already taken one step to improve the ability of your community's EMS system to save lives. You have increased the chances that a trained person — you — may be able to help at the scene of an accident or other medical emergency until EMS personnel arrive. Your ability to provide care immediately could save a life.

Components of an EMS System

Providing the victim with the right care at the right time is not an easy task. Although most communities have some way of sending medical help to victims of sudden illness or accidents, this help may not include everything that the victim needs and may not arrive in time to give the victim the best chance of surviving. Your community's ability to get the right help to the victim as quickly as possible requires both planning and resources. EMS systems that do this effectively usually have the following parts:

1. **Trained citizens** like you. Trained citizens can give first aid and alert the EMS system that a medical emergency has happened.

2. **Trained personnel.** To provide the best help quickly, an EMS system has specially trained personnel. These may include emergency medical technicians (EMTs), emergency medical technician-paramedics (paramedics), first responders (police, firefighters), emergency dispatchers, and hospital emergency department physicians and nurses trained in emergency medicine.

3. **Special equipment.** Different situations and medical needs require specialized medical, rescue, and transportation equipment.

4. **Communications systems.** How well the EMS system works depends on how quickly citizens can alert the system that an emergency has happened, and how quickly the dispatcher can get the appropriate emergency personnel to the scene. Communications systems are also important because EMS personnel often need to communicate with the hospital emergency department as they care for the victim at the scene of the emergency and on the way to the hospital.

5. **Management and evaluation.** An EMS system needs a management structure which includes administration and coordination of all parts of the system, medical supervision and direction, and ongoing evaluation and research.

The Responsibilities of the Rescuer in the EMS System

In order for the victim of a medical emergency to receive care from the EMS system, the victim must **enter** the system. This means that the EMS system must be told about the emergency and care should be given until EMS personnel arrive. These important first steps are generally performed by a citizen rescuer.

There are three things that **you** must do to make sure that a victim enters the EMS system with the best chance for survival:

1. **Recognize that a medical emergency has happened.** This isn't always easy. For example, you learned in Chapter 5 that victims of heart attack often deny that they are having a heart attack, making it difficult for bystanders to know something is wrong. Also, victims of accidents may be so concerned about the well-being of another injured person that they may not realize that they themselves are hurt. Medical problems are not always obvious, but the skills you have learned in this course will help you recognize emergencies.

2. **Give first aid (basic life support).** You have been trained to provide first aid for breathing and cardiac emergencies. CPR, rescue breathing, and first aid for choking are all basic life support techniques.

3. **Phone the EMS system for help.** You may phone or direct bystanders to phone for help. Give all necessary information so that appropriate medical care can reach the scene of the emergency. This information is discussed in Chapter 2.

How an EMS System Responds to a Call for Help

In many communities, a dispatcher will answer your call. The dispatcher is very important in making sure that the victim gets the right care immediately. In some systems, this person has special training to get specific information from the caller and to know which personnel and equipment to send to the scene. Some dispatchers can also give first aid instructions to the caller over the phone when it is necessary.

Basic Life Support and Advanced Life Support

As explained in Chapter 2, the information you provide to the EMS dispatcher is important. It will help determine the type of care that the dispatcher sends to the scene of an emergency. The dispatcher may send either an ambulance capable of continuing **basic life support,** or an ambulance capable of delivering **advanced life support.** The care sent will depend on the needs of the victim and the services available in your community.

Most requests for emergency medical services require basic life support. For this reason, many states require that all ambulances be staffed with personnel trained to provide at least basic life support.

Some requests for assistance also require advanced life support. For example, a victim of heart attack or cardiac arrest requires both basic life support and advanced life support. Advanced life support personnel may be supervised by a hospital-based physician.

A key thing to remember is that basic life support and advanced life support must be given within specific time periods in order to give the victim the best chance of survival. This is why it is important to have a well-coordinated EMS system in your community. Highly trained personnel can do more to help the victim if they arrive promptly.

Appendix — The Emergency Medical Services (EMS) System

First Responders

When a dispatcher receives a call for emergency medical help, the dispatcher will select the type of care that is needed and send the appropriate personnel. This may include police, fire, rescue, and ambulance personnel, depending on the type of emergency and the resources available at the time of the call.

In many communities, police and fire fighters may arrive at the scene before the ambulance because they are often located closer to the scene of the emergency. If you have been caring for a victim, the "first responder" may take over or ask you to assist. On the other hand, the first responder may tell you to continue care while he or she attends to other problems at the scene. It is important that you do not stop caring for a victim until the first responder takes over. You should expect the first responder to ask you for information about the victim. Information that you have gained from your primary and secondary surveys of the victim may be valuable to first responders, EMTs, paramedics, and to the hospital staff who will care for the victim later.

When the Ambulance Arrives

When the ambulance arrives, the EMTs or paramedics will take over responsibility for care of the victim and will provide additional medical care. Their goal is to begin to stabilize the victim's condition (correct life-threatening problems) at the scene. Once this has been done, the EMS personnel will prepare the victim for transport to the appropriate hospital emergency department, and they will continue caring for the victim on the way. When the ambulance arrives at the hospital, the EMS personnel will transfer responsibility for care of the victim to the emergency department staff.

You and Your EMS System

As you can see, the process by which you and the EMS system work together to save a life is complex. You should know that many communities do not have EMS systems that contain all of the features described above.

If you have ever been concerned about someone close to you having a heart attack or being the victim of a medical emergency, you owe it to yourself to find out what type of care your community's EMS system can provide in an emergency **before** an emergency happens. When minutes count, your knowledge of your community's EMS system can help you make the right decisions. The following checklist has been included to help you find out more about your community's EMS system.

A Guide to Assessing Your Community's Emergency Medical Services (EMS) System

The following questions reflect the EMS standards set forth in the Emergency Medical Services Systems Act of 1973, the federal EMS legislation.

1. Are regularly scheduled CPR and first aid classes, open to the public, offered in your community? YES _____ NO _____

2. Does your community have a 911 emergency number for EMS, fire, and police? YES _____ NO _____

3. Do your local schools certify students in first aid and CPR? YES _____ NO _____

4. Are local police officers trained and certified in American Red Cross First Aid or in the U.S. Department of Transportation First Responder training? YES _____ NO _____

5. Is your local ambulance service staffed by EMTs? YES _____ NO _____

6. Does your local ambulance service regularly leave the station to answer an emergency call within two minutes of receiving the call? YES _____ NO _____

7. Does your community have advanced life support units staffed by EMT-paramedics? YES _____ NO _____

8. Are rescue services in your community (EMS, police, fire) provided by well-equipped units staffed by EMTs? YES _____ NO _____

9. Are all emergency services in your community dispatched and coordinated through a central emergency communications center? YES _____ NO _____

10. Is your nearest hospital emergency department staffed on a 24-hour basis by physicians and nurses who are specially trained in emergency medicine? YES _____ NO _____

11. Does your community have a plan to transfer very acutely ill or injured patients to specialty centers? YES ____ NO ____

12. Does your community have an area-wide disaster plan to deal with multi-casualty incidents, natural disasters, and environmental emergencies? YES ____ NO ____

13. Is there one office in charge of the administration, coordination, and evaluation of the EMS system? YES ____ NO ____

Adapted from "A Community Scoring Guide for Emergency Health Services," Office of Emergency Medical Services, The Pennsylvania State University.

With a better idea of the different parts and responsibilities of a community emergency medical services system, you will be better able to assess the emergency medical services offered by your own community.

Your answers to the preceding questions will help you evaluate the services that your community provides. The questions to which you have answered YES will show you the strengths of your community's EMS system. The questions to which you have answered NO will point out areas where your community's EMS system could be strengthened. As a citizen and a taxpayer, your support of your community's EMS system is as important as your knowing how to perform first aid.

The American Red Cross

The American Red Cross is a name for people in your community who can help you prevent, prepare for, and cope with emergencies, whether those emergencies involve blood, disaster, health and safety, social services, or tissue transplants.

The Red Cross is nearly 1.5 million well-trained and dedicated volunteer and paid staff members who serve in every American community through some 2,900 chapters. Collectively, they are the largest volunteer service and educational force in the country. These individuals are supported by the skills and resources of a national organization. Together, they form the most effective and extensive emergency network in America—a network that extends to alleviate suffering here at home and around the world through the International Red Cross and Red Crescent Movement.

All these essential Red Cross services are made possible by the voluntary services, blood donations, and financial support of the American people.

Glossary

Abdominal Thrust — an upward thrust to the abdomen given to clear the airway of a person with a complete airway obstruction. Also called the **Heimlich maneuver.** *(Chapter 4)*

Air Exchange — the process of respiration or breathing; inhalation and exhalation of air into and out of the lungs. *(Chapter 4)*

Airway — the passageway through which air enters the body and goes to the lungs. *(Chapters 2, 3, and 4)*

Airway Obstruction — an obstruction or blockage of the airway that happens when the back of the tongue moves to block the airway, or the tissues of the throat swell. See **Mechanical Obstruction.** *(Chapter 3)*

Arteries — the blood vessels that carry blood from the heart to the cells of the body.

Artificial Respiration — see **Rescue Breathing.** *(Chapter 3)*

Blockage — see **Airway Obstruction** and **Mechanical Obstruction.**

Blood Pressure — the force of the circulating blood pushing against the walls of the blood vessels. *(Chapter 5)*

Blood Vessels — the tubes through which blood circulates throughout the body. *(Chapter 6)*

Breastbone — the bone at the front and center of the chest to which the ribs connect. *(Chapter 6)*

Breathlessness — the absence of breathing. *(Chapter 3)*

Cardiac Arrest — the condition when the heart stops beating; requires prompt CPR to keep blood flowing to the brain and cells of the body. *(Chapter 5)*

Glossary

CPR — the abbreviation for cardiopulmonary resuscitation. *(Chapter 6)*

Cardiac Emergency — a life-threatening condition when the heart is not functioning properly, such as during a heart attack or a cardiac arrest. *(Chapters 5 and 6)*

Cardiopulmonary Resuscitation (CPR) — an emergency procedure used for a person who is not breathing and whose heart has stopped beating (cardiac arrest). It is used to keep the body's cells from dying until advanced medical help arrives. The procedure involves a combination of rescue breathing and chest compressions. *(Chapter 6)*

Cardiovascular Disease — the disease characterized by the gradual clogging of blood vessels by fatty substances; associated with heart attack, stroke, high blood pressure, and diabetes. *(Chapter 1)*

Carotid Pulse — the beat which is felt at the side of the neck when the carotid artery is pressed. Located between the windpipe and the neck muscle, the carotid pulse is checked to determine the presence or absence of heartbeat. See **Pulse.**. *(Chapters 3 and 6)*

Chest Compression — a procedure for manually circulating blood in a person whose heart has stopped beating. It involves pressing up and down on the lower half of the breastbone. CPR is the combination of chest compressions and rescue breathing. *(Chapter 6)*

Chest Thrust — a thrust to the middle of the breastbone used to clear the airway. It is used for a person with complete airway obstruction who is extremely overweight or in the late stages of pregnancy. *(Chapter 4)*

Cholesterol — a fatty substance found in foods and also produced by the body. High levels of cholesterol in the body are associated with clogging of the blood vessels. *(Chapter 5)*

Circulatory System — the system that carries blood to all the cells of the body. Its main components are the blood vessels and the heart. *(Chapter 6)*

Complete Airway Obstruction — a condition in which a person is choking and completely unable to breathe, cough, or speak because something is blocking his or her airway. *(Chapters 3 and 4)*

Decontamination — a thorough cleansing to rid an object of germs and contaminants.

Disinfecting Solution — the liquid used to clean training manikins in order to prevent the spread of infectious diseases.

EMS — the abbreviation for emergency medical services.

EMS Dispatcher — a member of the emergency medical services system who receives emergency calls and coordinates sending the appropriate personnel and equipment to the scene of an accident or sudden illness. *(Chapter 2; Appendix, Emergency Medical Services System)*

Emergency Action Principles — the four basic steps to be followed in all emergency situations to ensure that victims receive proper care. *(Chapter 2)*

Emergency Medical Services (EMS) System — a community-based system that delivers specialized care for victims of injury or sudden illness. Care is provided at the scene of the emergency, and is continued during transportation and following arrival at an appropriately equipped health-care facility. *(Appendix, Emergency Medical Services System)*

Finger Sweep — a technique used as part of the procedure to dislodge and remove a piece of food or an object from the airway of an unconscious choking victim. *(Chapter 4)*

Head-tilt/Chin-lift — a technique used to open the airway of an unconscious person. It is performed by applying backward pressure to the forehead and lifting the jaw. This tilts the head back and lifts the chin. *(Chapter 3)*

Heart Attack — a condition in which blood flow to part of the heart is blocked, causing that part of the heart muscle to die because of lack of oxygen. *(Chapter 5)*

Heimlich Maneuver — see **Abdominal Thrust.**

Glossary

High Blood Pressure — a condition in which the pressure of the blood in the circulatory system is higher than normal. This condition is related to cardiovascular disease. *(Chapter 5)*

Implied Consent — a legal term used to describe the assumption that an unconscious person, if he or she were conscious, would have given consent to a rescuer to provide first aid. *(Chapter 2)*

Infectious Disease — a disease that can be transmitted or spread; a contagious disease.

Manikin — a life-size model of a person used for practicing first aid skills for respiratory and circulatory emergencies. *(Chapter 3)*

Mechanical Obstruction — obstruction or blockage of the airway caused by a piece of food or by a foreign object. *(Chapters 3 and 4)*

Mouth-to-Mouth Breathing — a form of rescue breathing during which a rescuer breathes air into the mouth and lungs of a person who is not breathing. *(Chapter 3)*

Mouth-to-Nose Breathing — a form of rescue breathing in which a rescuer breathes air into the nose and lungs of a person who is not breathing. This is done when injuries or other difficulties make it impossible to perform mouth-to-mouth breathing. *(Chapter 3)*

Mouth-to-Stoma Breathing — a form of rescue breathing in which a rescuer breathes air into the stoma and lungs of a person who is not breathing. *(Chapter 3)*

Nausea — a feeling of sickness in the stomach with an urge to vomit.

"Notch" — the place where the lower ribs meet the lower end of the breastbone in the center of the chest. Used as a reference point for finding the correct hand position in CPR. *(Chapter 6)*

911 — a special telephone number used in many communities to give fast, direct connection to police, fire, and emergency medical services.

Obstruction — blockage. See **Airway Obstruction.** *(Chapters 3 and 4)*

Oxygen — a gas that the cells of the body need in order to live. The air we breathe contains about 21 percent oxygen. *(Chapter 3)*

Oxygen-carrying Blood — blood that contains oxygen. *(Chapter 3)*

Partial Airway Obstruction — a partial blockage of the airway that allows some air exchange to occur. *(Chapters 3 and 4)*

Primary Survey — a series of checks to discover conditions that are immediately life threatening to a victim. *(Chapter 2)*

Pulse — the rhythmic "beat" in an artery. As the heart pumps blood, the walls of the arteries expand and contract, causing a beat or a pulse. This beat or pulse can be felt by pressing on an artery. *(Chapter 3)*

Rescue Breathing — the process of breathing air into the lungs of a person who has stopped breathing. Mouth-to-nose and mouth-to-stoma breathing are types of rescue breathing. Also called **Artificial Respiration.** *(Chapter 3)*

Rescuer — a person trained to survey the scene of an emergency, determine the extent of injuries, and provide first aid until EMS personnel arrive. *(Chapter 2)*

Respiratory Emergency — a condition where normal breathing is interrupted by an airway obstruction or other problem that interferes with normal breathing. *(Chapters 3 and 4)*

Respiratory System — the body system which draws air into the body and expels waste gases. The main components are the airway and the lungs. *(Chapter 3)*

Glossary

Resuscitation — an effort to restore to life. *(Chapters 3, 4, and 6)*

Risk Factors — conditions and behaviors that increase the likelihood of a person's developing a disease. Some risk factors (age, sex, race, and heredity) for cardiovascular disease cannot be changed. Others relate to life-style and can be changed. *(Chapter 5)*

Secondary Survey — a series of checks to discover conditions that are not immediately life threatening to a victim, but which may become life threatening if not corrected. These checks are done after life-threatening injuries have been found and cared for. *(Chapter 2)*

Stoma — a surgically created opening in the front of the neck through which a person breathes. *(Chapter 3)*

Stroke — a condition in which one or more of the blood vessels to the brain becomes clogged or bursts, causing a part of the brain to die from lack of oxygen. *(Appendix: Information About Stroke)*

Universal Distress Signal for Choking — action in which a choking victim grasps at his or her throat to signal that he or she is choking. *(Chapter 4)*

Unresponsiveness — a condition in which a person does not react to verbal or physical stimuli. *(Chapters 3, 4, and 6)*

Notes

Notes

Notes

Notes

Notes

Notes

Notes

Notes

Notes